Praise for *The Magic Eye*

"In *The Magic Eye*, Caryn Mirriam-Goldberg transforms the harrowing reality of a rare cancer diagnosis and the urgent fight to save a beloved fifth-generation farm into a luminous, poetic meditation on survival, community, and resilience. With tenderness and humor, her memoir speaks to the fierce beauty of holding on to life, to land, and to hope when the odds seem insurmountable. A deeply human story, this book is a testament to courage and the power of place that will stay with you long after you turn the final page."
   ~ Harriet Lerner, Ph.D. author of *The Dance of Anger* and
      Why Won't You Apologize?

"No endorsement can do justice to this vivid, lyric, wise, wry, compassionate, profoundly spiritual memoir of passage through some severe life trials. *The Magic Eye* is a microcosmic epic of unvaunting human triumph. Bursting with life in its myriad forms, this is a book to love and to share."
   ~ Stephanie Mills, author of *In Service of the Wild* and
      Epicurean Simplicity

"In this outstanding, beautifully written memoir, celebrated poet Caryn Mirriam-Goldberg tells two interweaving stories of redemption, healing, and courage, contrasting the struggle to save her life—following a diagnosis of eye cancer—with the fight to preserve her husband's ancestral land in Kansas. It's a riveting tale that will lift your heart and deepen your courage. I loved it."
   ~ Mark Matousek, author of *Lessons From an American Stoic:*
      How Emerson Can Change Your Life

"We're really in a struggle right now all over the planet, and we need stories like *The Magic Eye* to make us more attentive and mindful in asking how we place ourselves in right relations with all of creation. Caryn Mirriam-Goldberg's memoir embodies how we can shift our lens—finding new ways to see that we don't live among resources, we live among relatives. This memoir reminds us how, if we care for

the land, it cares for us. It also shows us how much our own healing is rooted in our healing of the earth."
    ~ Daniel Wildcat, author of *On Indigenuity: Learning the Lessons of Mother Earth*

"You might expect that a former Poet Laureate of Kansas would have a way with words. But with this narrative, you find yourself immersed in a world that transcends words to evoke a visceral feeling of life's fragility and transitory nature. Comforting connections with a community of caring souls and the natural environment in which Caryn Mirriam-Goldberg is grounded provides sustenance and relatable stories worthy of being shared."
    ~ Dave Kendall, Filmmaker and Media Anthropologist, Prairie Hollow Productions

"The Magic Eye is indeed so. Magic, not in the sense of the fantastical but in making meaning out of thick pain. Caryn has gifted us with a poly-ocular view of life, death, darkness, and light that is inspiring, guiding, and uplifting. This magic eye reveals a journey through love, loss, suffering, recovery and our shared humanity. She uses her mixed bag of inheritance to conjure up the impossible out of seemingly catastrophic events. This memoir takes us by the hand through the curvy roads of cancer and the unbendable spirit of a writer not afraid to take notes on the brokenness of a moment, to humorously interweave it into a lyricism that metabolizes pain. Most importantly, this memoir reminds us that our bodies 'are not islands, and even islands aren't separate from what surrounds and changes them over time.' Her unwavering commitment to saving land, which is also her way to save her body, and her fascination with naming turtles and feelings, gift us with a chance to connect our own lives with our common humanity. The sharpness of her lyricism opens the heart to the wisdom of 'cancer and treatment don't change who we are but rather reveal it.'"
    ~ Marianela Medrano, PhD, author of *Rooting* and other titles
"The body is a land and the land is a body. Caryn Mirriam-Goldberg tells a dramatic, compelling, compassionate story about her second

experience with cancer—an ocular melanoma—and her and her husband's journey to save the family land. Turtles play an important part; after all, it's turtles all the way down. Caryn's struggles through the difficulties of cancer treatment, coupled with tornados, people's comings and goings, and the pandemic, are inspiring. I loved this book and would recommend this book to anyone who struggles with the uncertainties of life, which is everyone. It's incredibly well-written, poetic even; a joy to read."

~ Lewis Mehl-Madrona, Associate Clinical Professor of Family Medicine, University of New England and author of *Coyote Healing: Miracles in Narrative Medicine*

"In *The Magic Eye,* Caryn Mirriam-Goldberg shows us how family, unforgettable friends, and the natural world knit together a net supporting her trip to ocular cancer-land and her efforts to save her family's farm. Caryn's story asks unwieldy questions about life and land ownership, while relishing the small, minute-by-minute gifts we get by living in this world. *The Magic Eye* shows us how a memoir can help us recognize ourselves better by doing what she does: recognizing the sacred and the everyday, which might be the same."

~ Louise Krug, author of *How to Explain: A Memoir*

"Realizing one's story is tied to the land, land that has witnessed our hardest and best moments, is so humbling and comforting. This is a brave memoir, exposing the strength and vulnerability of surviving through our relationships with the land. Caryn Mirriam-Goldberg shows us, as we care for the land, the land cares for us all."

~ Courtney Masterson, ecologist, educator, land steward, and executive director of Native Lands Restoration Collaborative, Inc.

"Caryn Mirriam-Goldberg's memoir reminds me of all the interconnections of our existence and the importance of recognizing the love that helps us heal. Not everyone can be cured, but everyone can be healed. As a physician I am concerned about the health of my patients and also about the health of my community and global environment. Only a poet with a deep sense of meaning and purpose could accomplish this feat of literary creation. It is a book that I will read, re-read, and share with my patients and their families."

~ Richard L. Deming, MD, FACR, FACRO, Medical Director, MercyOne Richard Deming Cancer Center and Founder, Above + Beyond Cancer

THE MAGIC EYE

SELECTED BOOKS BY CARYN MIRRIAM-GOLDBERG

Poetry:
How Time Moves: New & Selected Poems
Followin the Curve
Chasing Weather: Tornadoes, Tempests, and Thunderous Skies in Word & Image, with photographer Stephen Locke
Landed
Animals in the House
Reading the Body
Lot's Wife

Memoir & Nonfiction:
Everyday Magic: A Field Guide on the Mundane and Miraculous
Poem on the Range: A Poet Laureate's Love Song to Kansas
Needle in the Bone: How a Holocaust Survivor and Polish Resistance Fighter Beat the Odds and Found Each Other
The Sky Begin At Your Feet: A Memoir on Cancer, Community and Coming Home to the Body

Fiction:
Miriam's Well
The Divorce Girl

Anthologies Edited:
Transformative Language Arts in Action, co-edited with Ruth Farmer
To the Stars Through Difficulties: A Kansas Renga in 150 Voices
The World Keeps Turning Toward Light: A Renga from the State Poets Laureate of America
Begin Again: 150 Kansas Poems
An Endless Skyway: Poems from the State Poets Laureate of America, co-edited with Walter Bargen, Denise Low & Marilyn K. Taylor
The Power of Words: A Transformative Language Arts Anthology, co-edited with Janet Tallman

THE MAGIC EYE

A Story of Saving a Life and a Place
in the Age of Anxiety

Caryn Mirriam-Goldberg

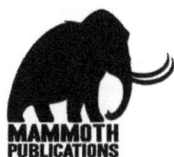

MAMMOTH
PUBLICATIONS

Mammoth Publications
Mammothpublications.net
610 Alta Vista Dr., Healdsburg, CA 95448

Earlier versions of some of this material appeared as "Everyday Magic"
blog posts on CarynMirriamGoldberg.com.

Cover Photo: Selfie by Caryn Mirriam-Goldberg
Book Design: Paul Hotvedt

ISBN: 978-1-939301-57-4
Library of Congress Control Number: 2025905008

To all the aunties who made saving a place possible and made my life so much more loving, especially Wilma, Eleanor, Rhoda, and Jill

Contents

III
THE GATES ARE NEVER CLOSED

Introduction
HOW I GOT HERE

All I knew when I first walked this land was that Ken, my new boy-friend, had lost his brown wallet in the brown dirt. It was twilight, and Ken, his dad Gene, and I walked the horizontal ruts between the rows Ken just plowed. Just when we were about to give up, I looked down to-ward something square and brown and found it, half-buried in the soft dirt. I didn't know that September 1983 day how searching for treasure in that dirt would become a lifetime occupation.

Close to forty years later, I step barefoot onto the back deck of the house we built here. It's a cold April morning, the air just above freezing as I walk carefully to avoid some of the nails that weather has shimmied out of the wood planks. Like most days, I head to the western edge of the deck for a better view of the land we have spent all these years trying to save without knowing how much it was saving us.

To the west, low-lying fog holds the prairie we replanted, with reddened big bluestem and switch grass fallen over, exhausted by freeze and thaw of early spring. If I cover my left eye, my right eye, damaged by cancer and radiation, sees a watercolor of dark green cedar rows dissolving into the pale blue of sky. Both eyes and the rest of me are continually learning to see where I live, impossibly fraught in a tangle of wounded ownership for decades that made it, like this body, vulner-able to invasion and destruction. What happened was both incremental and sudden, wave and particle, fate and liminal.

Both this land and I are fortunate survivors, against the odds. I've tunneled through cancer twice while living in and with this place. This land has made it through its own seemingly impossible story despite so many beloved places just like this lost to bulldozers, generational trauma, and the lure of big dollars.

Since the mid-1980s, Ken and I tried—argued, wrote, researched, reasoned, cried, talked, prayed, and planned—to save the 130 acres that his family has inhabited for over 150 years. If there were statistical analyses for survival rates for land (like there often are for cancer), surely this land would have been given only a one to two percent chance of not being plowed and subdivided, something I'm reminded of when I look all four directions.

To the north, there's Lawrence, Kansas, with a consistently hot and bothered real estate market, and businesses that can sell you vegan Pad Thai, a mermaid tattoo, a cow-shaped lamp, books on deep ecology and overcoming racism, or a latte with a perfectly-drizzled sleeping cat on the foam. Yet Lawrence still has small town touches, like the city band playing a medley from, obviously, *The Wizard of Oz* in South Park before an audience of oldsters in lawn chairs and tutu-bedecked five-year-olds twirling on the grass

To the west, the emboldened blue sky frames the highway that we fought against to prevent the destruction of native prairies, tribal burial grounds, and historic ruts from the Santa Fe trail. Working with a coalition of fourth- and fifth-generation farmers, free spirits, history buffs, native people fiercely protecting (yet again) hidden sacred sites, and people in love with tallgrass prairies, we won a half victory. The highway proceeded, but not on a path that would have destroyed much of what we sought to save.

To the south, controlled fires burn. For over a year a developer has been burning acres of cedars, Osage orange trees, prairie grasses, and brome fields to make way for dozens of suburban houses. This could easily have been the fate of our land.

To the east, less than an hour's drive, there's the Kansas City metro with historic theaters boosting jazz singers or stand-up comics, the world-class Nelson Atkins Museum of Art, many manner of teams worth obsessing over (the Royals, the Chiefs), big box stores selling the usual stuff, and tiny shops pitching up-cycled clothing or motorcycle detailing.

For half of Ken's life, the lion's share of the farm belonged to his grandfather, Bill Wells. By the time I met Bill, he had mellowed . . . .sort of—Ken and I, not a couple yet, stopped by his Topeka house on our way back to Lawrence. "When I see that," Bill said pointing to my Carter Mondale bumper sticker, "I want to get my shotgun and shoot it off."

"When I see that," I said, pointing to the Regan bumper sticker on his front storm door, "I want to get your shotgun and shoot it off."

His face broke into a huge smile, showing me his missing and remaining teeth, and from then on, he accepted me as part of the pack because I didn't cower. I didn't know if I would see him again, but having been raised by a similar kind of man, I knew bullies only respected strength, and humor didn't hurt (although I had no idea how to use a shotgun). Bill didn't buy that I wasn't Ken's girlfriend either.

Passing on land owned by one person to more than one heir is often messy, but infinitely so when Bill willed the land to the five daughters he abandoned in 1937. According to family legend, when his wife Forrest Elizabeth gave birth to a fifth daughter, he said, "Not another damn girl," then left their small two-bedroom house made from limestone quarried from the top of the hill.

He stayed away for years, sent iffy to no child support. He married and divorced and remarried. Eventually he made strides to rebuild relationships with some of his daughters, leaving behind a legacy of vastly-imperfect love by giving them this land. His daughters, all well past middle-age by the time he died, put the land in a rarified trust that gave each of them equal and undivided interest. This prevented any moves, from selling the whole thing to dividing up parcels, without unanimous agreement.

Some would say he gave them this land—like most land, carrying buried layers of promises and betrayals—as a peace offering. Others speculated it was a mean-spirited ploy to tear his family apart. I think of the inheritance as a hybrid apology, blessing, hope, and legacy buried in sedimentary wounds and ruptures. Whether the inheritance was meant as a gift or a burden, it quickly turned into a problem that was insoluble, with no clear way to even talk about, let alone figure out what to do with the land. As the Wells sisters aged, some right out of this life, the problem grew more fraught.

Whatever we inherit is usually a mixed bag. At my mom's 80th birthday, as I was thanking her for passing on her love of art and books as well as a passion for peace and women's rights, I also had to add two more things: anxiety and cancer. Our bodies are shaped and infused by health practices and promises (broken and kept), wrong turns, and joyful mistakes, not to mention genetics, history, time, and environment. But where else can we live than here in our bodies, our most local addresses?

Yet bodies are not islands, and even islands aren't separate from what surrounds and changes them over time. We live on what seems to be islands of property, but all are part of a larger body of earth, which lives in the body of sky. Measuring beginnings of the earth is often like drawing a circle around a bobbing spot in the ocean, soon to smooth out or rush the beach to disappear itself. But dates can serve as placeholders, especially looking back: April 30, 2019, for my diagnosis of eye cancer at the age of 59, March 13, 2020, for when the pandemic hit home, and December 15, 2020, for when Ken and I signed a stack of papers to buy this land where we've lived since January 1, 1996. Saying when this story started is like naming the beginning of a full moon rising behind trees, buildings, ridges, and highways that block its glow. You know it's out there, behind the cloud cover, yet how did it start?

Back in 1982, I met Ken at the first Kansas Area Watershed (KAW) Council gathering, a newly- formed bioregional group rooted in deep ecology and branching into a pack of people spending our evenings together at meetings, potlucks, and events of our own creation. I was 22, he was 27, and both of us were finding our sea legs again after difficult break-ups. First we were friends, then a year later, each other's rebounds. Neither of us felt the pressure to believe a little fling would flourish. But it did.

While looking for Ken's wallet a year after we met, I didn't yet know that while Ken was and still is prone to lose anything in his pockets (wallets, keys, cell phones, screwdrivers, pocketknives), he was a genius at not losing this farm.

I was a genius at not losing the sky. I tracked it well back before I had words, between New York city buildings and long arms of trees reaching for where they ended and the blue began. Having grown up in tight Brooklyn apartments, then a triplex in East Flatbush, I was amazed when we moved to a Manalapan, New Jersey, suburb to discover bigger views from our house on top of a hill, especially from my bedroom window.

Our family, broken and breaking just as the woodlands cleared for these Levitt houses, was riddled with loud fights and smashed Hummel figurines. This propelled me to look for a place to belong. From narrow city streets to wider suburban lanes, I was always falling in love with clouds wheeling into shapes as well as hard-lit blue clearings.

The sky was especially elusive all those Saturdays and holidays I spent in my dad's underground stamp store (for collectors and investors) in the Nassau-Fulton subway arcade of lower Manhattan. I would climb up the blackened cement steps as the heat from the subway poured upward—the smell of home to me—and look up. There the sky was in the slits I could make out between tops of tall buildings. I loved the city, which I wandered on my own as a nine-year-old, but I loved the sky more.

Without knowing any farmers or farms beyond Delicious Orchards in central Jersey, where we bought apple pies and cider donuts, I dreamt of living on a farm. The dream didn't include actual farming, as foreign to me as becoming an astronaut, especially the pre-dawn wake-ups, 14-hour days, and low profits, if any. But as a city girl with a passion for open space, such romantic notions die hard.

Even the death, when I was ten, of my brother, Jeffrey Todd, from SIDS, was an event of sky proportions. It was raining hard until it wasn't. Then something I had never seen before, although surely it must have been in plain view had I known where to look: a rainbow. "This is what God gave us for taking away the baby," my grandmothers, crying in Yiddish, translated to me.

Despite another sister being born a year later, my family's tenuous hold as a nuclear unit exploded apart. Even the houseplants, wandering Jews spilling out of macrame hangers (it was the '70s), died after my father poured Ivory Liquid into each to hurt my mother. But when a judge asked who I wanted to live with, I chose my father because that seemed the best way to stay in the house where I experienced occasional rainbows.

What followed was insult and injury from my parent of choice. I wore my bruises to high school, hiding the latest under wraps. No wonder that having already been primed to make things—I was a kid artist from the time I could hold a fat red crayon—I turned to poetry as my saving grace. But what my poetry was always about, is still about, is the earth and sky.

The dirt, the smell of the air after a May rain or the storm gathering on the horizon, had always been a godsend for me. I hid in the hill behind our house, out of reach of my father's words or slaps, in an overgrown jungle of whatever grew on its own, journal in hand. I yearned to live somewhere with big views and with someone who loved me, a dream that seemed as unreachable as my fantasies of winning an Academy Award as I ran down a suburban sidewalk, my arms spread and acceptance speech already memorized.

"I'm going to live in Kansas one day," I announced to my maternal grandfather, Papa, when I was five. He reminded me of this, laughing in his Polish accent, just after Ken and I married.

Marrying Ken in 1985 meant marrying a farm too. Ken worked alongside his grandfather from boyhood, raising corn, soybeans, milo, oats, wheat, and alfalfa until changing economics and woodland invasions made farming unsustainable. Because of Ken's work on the farm—from chasing truant chickens to putting in many hours in the grime and heat of fixing old tractors and other farm equipment—his grandfather deeded him five acres for a future home.

In 1986, Ken began managing the farm for the family, focusing on turning about twenty-five acres into native plants of the tallgrass prairie, which means burning it each spring to keep the soil healthy and the invader cedars at bay. We have raised no livestock, although this land teems with deer, coyotes, raccoons, possums, rabbits, snakes, wild turkeys, occasional bobcats and foxes, and a whole flyway of birds cycling through from the Gulf of Mexico to the Arctic and back each year.

We had matching dreams of building a house on this land, me with my old sky love and Ken with his honed passion for astronomy and weather. In the early 1990s, we wandered the land, initially planning on a home nestled against the woods on the east side of the hill. But one winter day rounding the western flank of the hill on our way back to the car, we found another place. Close to the woods, it faced southwest to whatever weather was parading through—storms of gymnastic clouds or clear-skied easy strolls. We sat on the grass and watched the sky.

"Is this it?" I asked.

"Yup," he answered.

In 1994, we thought we were building a house for our foursome of a family—Ken, me, Daniel born in 1989, and Natalie in 1992—but after we broke ground, we found we were to be five. Forest was born five months after we moved into the house. We didn't change our design— passive solar, angled to work in concert with the sky—but we did make one closet bigger.

Along the way, Ken went from a degree in anthropology, which translated into making tofu for a living, to going back to school to become an occupational therapist, so he could work with people who live with disabilities. I worked long hours for minimal pay as a grassroots organizer on energy and labor issues before going back to school to study poetry, where I discovered I had a twin calling in teaching. By the time we moved to the new house, I was a graduate teaching assistant at the University of Kansas finishing a PhD in poetry.

The house was one dream, but there was a bigger dream that held the house. When we got married we vowed that we would buy or otherwise find a way to protect all of his family's original land holdings. It turned out that the quote we used in our wedding ceremony from Wendell Berry would also be the story of marrying this land:
The meaning of marriage begins in the giving of words. We cannot join ourselves to one another without giving our word. And this must be an unconditional giving, for in joining ourselves to another we join ourselves to the unknown. We can join one another only by joining the unknown. We must not be misled by the procedures of experimental thought: in life, in the world, we are never given two known results to choose between, but only one result that we choose without knowing what it is.
We couldn't know what we were getting into, but we were heart-bent on going.

We also couldn't know all else the land would give us. Here was where we found refuge during my first cancer, invasive breast cancer. When my father died, then Ken's father, then Ken's mother, and so many dear friends, some by surprise and some slowly over time, the land was this place full of bird song that sustained and healed us.

Time passed, and I remain settled in one place: After each child started school, then college, then whatever confusing path showed itself. After each drive to town to refill five-gallon jugs with drinkable water because our well water was too salty from remnants of old oceans. After each long or short work trip or family reunion or exciting-at-first and exhausting-in-the-end family vacation camping in the mountains with altitude sickness and teenage attitude. After taking in an abandoned dog and several cats who just showed up at our home, and years later after their expected or unexpected deaths, burying our beloved pets near the garden. After we drove used cars into the ground, then sold each to buy another used car to drive as long as it would go. After all this, it was the view of the sky and walks through the land—carefully and quickly during chigger and tick season, with dogs still alive or just gone—that restored us as we aged. It was this land, a perch in the cosmos, a still point in the big winds of each storm and the clearing afterwards, that owned us.

I

NAMING THE TURTLES

1

Naming the Turtles

Throughout it all, I've been naming turtles.

It started when Ben, a young shaggy-banged professor at Washburn University in Topeka, showed up at our front porch holding a beautiful large female turtle. He had heard we loved turtles, so here he was. When I asked for her name, he said all the turtles were numbered instead. "She's so gorgeous that she should have a name made of letters, not just numbers," I told him. He agreed. I named her Lucille thinking both of Lucille Ball because this turtle had orange flecks and the Kenny Rogers' song with the chorus, "You picked a fine time to leave me, Lucille." He pasted a turtle-sized transmitter on Lucille's back, then drove her back to one of his many sites in northeast Kansas to release her and find more turtles. Because Ben is a turtle whisperer, he's kept me busy.

That was in the summer of 2018, and the next spring, he re-found Lucille as well as Samantha, Theodore, and the three-toed box turtle I named Rudolph. Lately, because of heavy rains, he found a bumper crop of new turtles for me to name.

I spend a lot of time surrounded by indoor animals too. There was Shay, a labaraner (chocolate lab and Weimaraner mix) who showed up also at our front door, starving and sick on a freezing February morning. Miyako, a four-and-a-half pound Velcro kitty, wanted to be held 24/7 and mainly lived on love. Daniel found Sidney Iowa, an abandoned kitten on a 104-degree day when he traveled with friends Courtney and Denise to Sidney, Iowa, so they could get legally married (before gay marriage was legal in America). This herd—two black-and-white tabbies and one horse-like dog—have ferried me from porch to living room, stood guard at the bathroom door, and escorted me to the front door if I was planning to leave without them. Because Shay, with his long, elegant dog fingers, could both open the fridge and turn on the stove's gas burners, we had to child-proof everything in the kitchen long after our human offspring had moved out.

On April 28, 2019, while Ben was searching for turtles at area farms, I was driving to the ophthalmologist to find out why my right eye was seeing things out of focus. I had only paid attention to the right eye acting up because my pal Jules, in her Memphis accent, had recently asked over lunch, "What's up with your eye? It keeps twitching." We were catching up at a fast clip over the best cauliflower soup in the world at one of our favorite restaurants. Our large glasses of iced tea made us talk faster as we downed salad and jumbo shrimp before splitting an apple tart. Maybe I just needed new glasses, I mused, but I promised her I'd go to a doctor.

Dr. Sandal, an integrative medicine physician I'd been seeing to boost my health from long-term after-effects of chemo, examined my eye carefully with a tiny light while having me look various directions. He didn't have the equipment to do more, but he wondered if I just had an infection in my cheek. No big deal, but just to be sure, he made an appointment with the first ophthalmologist with an opening.

Now I was walking up the white-painted cinderblock stairway of a medical arts building to the office of Dr. George Jones, so I could get an answer. Never mind that I was an Olympic-medal-placing worrier (I also placed silver in rumination), especially about health issues. There's nothing like one cancer diagnosis even in a family full of diagnoses—my father, uncle, aunt, and step-father all died from pancreatic cancer, my mother and aunt had each had breast cancer twice—to turn a tension headache into worry about a brain tumor. But since I didn't know eye cancer was a thing, I didn't know how to freak out.

I sat obediently in the waiting room, returning some emails on my laptop until it was time to have my eye examined. The technician, a kind and efficient young woman with a strawberry-blonde ponytail and black-rimmed glasses, dilated my eyes and had me look various directions. Then Dr. Jones, a tall glass of water with curly hair and green eyes, surely not much older than my son Daniel, sat on a rolling stool and had me look through a phoropter, a metallic mosaic of cylinders, prisms and lenses that measures the eyes and their vision.

He got quieter as we went on, and my worries started trotting, then galloping. "Could it be glaucoma?" I asked although I didn't really know what that was, only that it sounded deliciously like guacamole. "No," he told me. "Cataracts?" I wondered, dreading having to deal with another surgery. Not that either, he assured me but also anti-assured me with his silence. "We need more tests, but it's definitely something," he said.

I was whisked to another room where I had to sit very still looking through various peepholes in machines that were imagining my peepers from many angles. Half an hour later, I was back in the examination room.

Dr. Jones came in and scooted his stool so close that his face was only about a foot from mine. He batted his long lashes while holding his mouth in a line of concern. I had my notebook and pen out, having learned long ago the value of writing down everything at such moments if, for no other reason, the movement of my hand over the page gave me some sense of agency.

"There's serious damage to the right eye," he began. "It could be a metastasis. Actually, there's a good chance it's a melanoma."

I just stared at him, such a strong sensation of falling overtaking me that I thought I might speed-slump out of the comfortable examination seat.

"It's cancer," he said softy. "A tumor." He leaned in a little more, his green eyes looking into my green ones.

"Wait, let me call Ken and put him on speaker phone," I answered, never having planned to hear such a diagnosis alone. Ken didn't answer despite a few attempts, so I asked Dr. Jones to go on.

"It's probably just an ocular melanoma, something that can be easily treated. They can either do radiation treatments, or the more likely treatment would be a radiative implant that would clear it up. You could lose an eye. Or," he said, going quieter, "it could be a metastasis from somewhere else."

I've been an inhabitant in Cancer World for enough years to know exactly what he was saying: brain tumor or something else dauntingly terminal-sounding. But my survival instinct must have poured a numbing agent through my bloodstream because I heard myself, from a long distance off, ask in a higher-pitched voice than normal, "It's treatable?"

"Completely," he said without telling me treatable didn't necessarily mean curable. Of course that was only if it was a melanoma, and even then, it would have to be a treatable melanoma. Still, my body knew terror when it smelled it in a small, dim office with shiny equipment ready to do its job.

I stumbled out of the chair, as Dr. Jones worked with the receptionist to get me an appointment with Dr. Komal Desai, the only ocular oncologist within hundreds of miles. I finally reached Ken, crying a little and barely able to say "Cancer, tumor, eye, come now." I called Dr. Sandal, and his nurse said to come over at noon, which was in twenty minutes. Ken raced the thirty miles from Topeka to Lawrence and later told me he was rehearsing what to say to highway patrol if they pulled him over for going 90 mph, something like "My wife is freaking out," although his pedal to the metal was his way of freaking out too.

When I heard Dr. Jones urgently whisper to the receptionist that June 2 was too far away for Dr. Desai to see me, my heart picked up its pace. "We'll be in touch," the receptionist called after me as I turned for the door. I managed to aim myself down the stairs, careful not to trip and hurt myself, sobbing in the echo chamber of the sterile stairwell.

I drove the three blocks to Dr. Sandal's office, and it not being time yet, called Kelley, one of my besties, while I paced the parking lot. What did I say to her? All I knew, through choking sobs. What did she say? All she could to hold me together, but I can't remember actual words. I only felt gravel under my shoes as I walked in circles, crying so much it was hard to speak or hear. Later I would joke with her about how the doctor had the same name of the country singer who belted out such hits as "If Drinkin' Don't Kill Me" and more fittingly, "The Cold Hard Truth." The blossoming trees all around soothed and mocked me at once. Kelley told me she loved me, I would get through this, but all I heard was the roar of panic revving its engines. The pebbles in the gravel parking lot glistened in the sun, and the air was unduly dry and sweet.

Then Ken and I were in Dr. Sandal's office, sitting across from him as he leaned forward, telling us we didn't have necessary information yet. We didn't know enough to flip out, but such thinking had never stopped me before. I wrote notes furiously in an effort to be the recorder of events and not the one living them. "We don't want to jump to any negative conclusions," Dr. Sandal said. As always, he hugged me goodbye, said to call anytime, said he would be there for us.

Walking back to the car, Ken put his arm around my shoulders and looked straight ahead. I glanced up at him and read the worry in his eyes. His just-turning-gray hair would soon turn much grayer. It was hard to believe but believe it we did as a sense of horror flooded our throats.

In search of sandbags to stop the surge, we drove to Pine's Garden Center to buy flowers to plant because, although I wasn't sure that would help, as goes the old Jewish joke about giving a dead man an enema, "It couldn't hurt." Before we got out of the car, Dr. Sherri Soule, my regular oncologist, returned a call I had forgotten I left for her. I put her on speaker phone while she and I made tentative plans to send me to the University of Iowa Medical Center, over five hours away. A world-class eye disease teaching hospital, this med center might be able to get me in much sooner than Dr. Desai.

As I stared at the gently swaying branches of a cottonwood tree, the obnoxious blue sky played its perpetual happy song, In the office, I heard Dr. Soule explain what was likely next: a PET scan to make sure the cancer was only in the eye. An MRI of my head to ensure no other cancer had metastasized from elsewhere to the brain. Both of us were speaking in code about breast cancer, so she quickly stopped to reassure me: "It's very rare for breast cancer to metastasize to the eye."

"How many eye cancers have you seen in your practice?" I asked, no pun intended.

"Only two in fifteen years. It's pretty rare," she answered. I tried to slow my breath.

"How did they turn out?"

She was quiet. "One was fine." We breathed on other ends of the phone. "I'm here for you," she said after a few beats.

Driving home, I began responding to phone calls. I cursed with Kris and lamented the news with Judy. Kris was a daily check-in friend, both of us working from home and up-to-date with all the nuances of our workaday challenges. We also took wandering day trips, heading out whatever direction on empty Kansas highways that inevitably led us to antique stores in falling-down barns and fried chicken in small-town cafes. Judy I've known for decades, and when I had breast cancer, which coincided with her sabbatical as a math professor at the University of Kansas, she made attending all my treatment sessions her project. Whatever balanced in her from being both a New York Jew and a Zen master funneled out in a steady ability to be present, funny, and able to abide with whatever painful news came crashing ashore.

I also called my mother, herself a triple cancer survivor. I tried to sound more cheerful than I was, as if this was a bad flu that would pass, but I could hear the concern in her voice. I would know more soon, I told her, cringing at what I might discover. My mom could be calm and quiet, or nervous and quiet, but she led with love and laughter.

Somewhere in the mix, Dr. Jones's receptionist called back. Dr. Desai would see us tomorrow, so sudden for a doctor with a full schedule that I got scared all over again. Walking into the house, carrying the new flowers—sweet Williams because they smelled good—we decided not to tell our kids until after we got the report from the doctor the next day. After all, they went through the fear wringer of the first cancer, and they didn't need to be overwhelmed with this one before we had the necessary information.

Meanwhile, there was this evening ahead of us of phone calls and flower-planting, rustling up something to eat and eating it, finding a funny distraction to watch on Netflix, and clutching each other as we slept before I turned away, too afraid to touch another human. I prayed myself to sleep with one word: *please.*

On the way to meet Dr. Desai, I named three more turtles—Demeter, Persephone, and Priscilla—a trio of goddesses. Then we drove in a rush-hour traffic to her office in Kansas City's St. Luke's Medical Center while I called Ravi, my brother, although we had different parents and grew up in different countries. I apologized for not calling him earlier, but since he lived in Kansas City, I wondered if he wanted to join us. "Of course," he said.

From the Sabates Eye Center waiting room, where televised women played tennis and women around us perused eye glass frames, we waited together, trying to be a cheery trio. Surely this would be a small fixable thing, like a new screw that needed to be added to a lawnmower to get it going again. I remember feeling the same way when I first heard the words "breast cancer," imagining surgery, a bit of radiation, then I'd be on my way. Of course, what happened was nothing like that.

We were called back to a small dark room where the technician dilated my eyes, then escorted me to an inner sanctum of another waiting room where on a television, a house rehab show drew the attention of others there waiting for the blur to overtake their eyes. "You nervous?" I asked Ravi. He nodded, and we tried to look at the news on our phones, check Facebook and email, get through the waiting.

Dr. Desai is a beautiful Indian woman, a decade or two younger than me, with large brown eyes, a long ponytail, and a face that communicates immense intelligence. I had a long list of questions, having been primed to chat extensively to learn all I could from my previous oncologists. "I heard it could be treated easily," I said, trying to sum up whatever I imagined Dr. Jones said yesterday.

"Who told you that?" she frowned. I tried to explain what Dr. Jones said, but she remained skeptical. Then after looking at my eye—having me aim my eyes down, down to the right, up to the right, down to the left, and so on—she said something that rattled all our bones.

"It's either a brain tumor or a good-sized melanoma."

"A brain tumor from my previous breast cancer?" I asked.

She nodded, not having to tell me that if a brain tumor was affecting my eye, it was already out of control, although what brain tumor is in control?

"Well, let's just root for the ocular melanoma," I said, trying to sound cheerful.

"They're both bad!" she answered.

Two-and-a-half years later, Ken said, "You were trying to make light of it, and she wasn't having any of it."

"But what was it like for you?" I asked.

"It was one of the worst moments of my life."

You think the bottom falls out once, then you regroup and go on, but it's a series of falling out bottoms, each one sending me lurching toward a bathroom to pee even if I barely had to go. But then I've learned intense fear can do that, make the body evacuate all it's holding in in preparation to fight the lurking enemy or run very fast and far away.

I already knew that the distance between potentially lethal news and the actual diagnosis is exponential, one number times another number times an infinity of fear. We went back to the tennis-on-TV waiting room. Ken, Ravi, and I sat in a row. I had just been through a number of tests, ones I would end up repeating dozens of times over the years to come.

For the first test, a dye was injected in my right arm, then I looked into a peep hole, trying to focus on what looked like the burning eye of Mordor (later this image was replaced by the logo for Walmart, which made sense to our family since whenever we passed a Walmart for years, we called out, "The fires of Mordor burn bright"). For another, I lay on a table while Phil—the tall gray fox of a technician I would see many times after this—slid a small cushion-ended pen over my eyeball for an ultrasound. With my eye already numb, it was actually a little relaxing, although I had to work hard to look down toward my feet, something a little discombobulating while lying down.

Now we were waiting for the results. I leaned my right shoulder into Ravi. "Do you think it's bad?"

He took off his glasses and rubbed his large brown eyes, then looked at me. "Yes," he answered, already crying. My heart sank. He thought I was going to die, and that thought was utterly convincing at this moment, but then I knew him well enough to know he could never have lied to me about what he was thinking. Ravi, whom I met folk-dancing in the early '80s, had always felt like family. In the course of getting to know him—from our salad days of him teaching me the Swedish hambo, the Romanian dance, Floricica Olteneasca, and more—that sense of being related deepened, but mostly through dreams we had when apart. We had years together of leaping and stomping our feet in Slavic dancing and leaping and twirling in Scandinavian ones.

"I dreamt I was you and married to Ken as I woke up and looked for my glasses, which were your glasses," he once told me. "But it wasn't bad at all to be married to Ken."

"I dreamt you and I were brothers crossing a big desert on camels," I had told him as he nodded.

When I met his mother, who came from Madras (now Chennai), India, to visit, she took to me like one of her kids. She nodded know-ingly at whatever I said while we drank tea, talked about redbirds in the tree, and understood why it was good that Ravi came here to do a PhD in chemical engineering after first planning on becoming pharmacist. From that point on, he never had a conversation with her when she didn't ask, "How is that Jewish girl?"

Now we were here in this waiting room, Ravi was still reeling from the death of the other person in his life who felt like family, a tango dance teacher named Toi, who was like his sister, teacher, partner, and best friend all at once. She died suddenly in his arms from a heart attack triggered by chronic obstructive pulmonary disease, and the bottom of his life fell out.

I got up to pace back and forth, calling some friends about what was happening, everyone reminding me that this waiting was the worst. I tried to breathe slowly even as I wanted to jump out of my skin, but seriously, where is there to go?

"It's an ocular melanoma," Dr. Desai said, but before I could cozy into relief, she added that the extreme possibilities were still extremely dire, and we wouldn't know for sure if the rest of the body was clear until after the PET scan of my torso and the MRI of my brain. Then we might find out if it was treatable. If it was, we'd begin.

"Wait, why are you writing this down? We'll give you medical records."

"She has to write everything down," Ken said.

"She's a writer. She can't help it," Ravi added.

Dr. Desai explained the tumor was five millimeters thick and drew me a picture of what looked like a small lopsided volcano. She moved to the screen where I saw what she drew in technicolor, a green universe with a dark secret growing more dangerous every day. We were stunned at how large the tumor was, so much so that it was impinging on blood vessels in my eye, which was why my vision was blurred. With treatment, I should get some vision back.

"Back?" I asked, suddenly hopeful I was going to live. I couldn't bear to look at Ken or Ravi, who I knew were spun in a freakout of epic proportion and surely hyperventilating in the corner where they sat.

Brachytherapy, a radiation treatment, was the way to go: a small gold disk with tiny seeds of radiation, each one a prayer for life, would be sewn into the disk and implanted in my eye. Five days of me being radioactive, enough that if the levels were too high I wouldn't be able to leave the hospital, a possibility that catapulted me back into losing my breath for a moment. Two surgeries Dr. Desai would do to put the disk in and taking it out, and in between, I would wear a lead shield over my eye and need to stay a big distance away from any humans or animals.

But I wanted to know more than I could write in my journal. What kind of gold? What was the shape? Did they sew it onto my eyeball? Dr. Desai patiently explained it was like a gold button with little eyelets around the edges where the radiation was sewn in. It had to be made out of town and shipped here. Would I have migraines from the treatment? How long would it take to recover? Is this tumor medium sized or big or humongous? What causes this? Mostly, will I live, will I live, will I live?

She answered everything, including the daunting numbers: there was a 30-50% chance that the cancer could spread, and if so, it was 90% likely to go to the liver. I coughed and gulped at once. "But there are promising trials to treat metastases." I knew enough from leading writing workshops for eighteen years for people with cancer and other illnesses to understand that "trials" often meant an extension of life, a remission of the cancer if all went well, and barring a miracle, numbered days ahead.

Micro-metastases were the biggest danger. I pictured tiny sparks from a distant fire. Melanomas are aggressive and eye ones even more so, but we would be monitoring everything. CT scans or MRIs every three months. For at least a decade. But for now, the next steps: all the scans and prep, the surgeries, the recovery. Then the healing. Then seeing what vision I had left. Then the aftermath which, I didn't know at the time, would lead to waves of dominos falling in the grand game of being a body.

We went home, putting whatever she said about dire possibilities out of mind. As we turned from I-35 onto Highway 10 to head west, I shut off NPR news and called my mother. "Wait, I'll shut off the news," she said, laughing a little about whatever mishegoss was happening in this messed-up world now. She laughed often all the time, a good counter-balance to whatever the world was ladling out.

"So we're driving home from Kansas City where we just saw an ocular oncologist because it turns out," I paused and looked at Ken. "I have a little melanoma, cancer, in my right eye." I didn't tell her it was actually more of a big melanoma.

She went silent, both of us thinking at the same time that I had already done my cancer time and shouldn't have this also, but then again, my mother had breast cancer twice and colon cancer once, so we knew better.

I explained the details in a jaunty way: scans to make sure I was fine otherwise, and I was sure I was, then the tiny gold disk going in to kill the cancer dead. "I'm sure it's going to be okay" repeatedly as much for her as for me, and then I asked her to call my sisters and brother for me and to let Aunt Rhoda, her sister, know. The phone calls would help her digest this and take some of the telling-the-story-as-if-it's-true pressure off of me a little bit.

"Okay, Pussycat," she said before we hung up. She hadn't called me Pussycat since I was a little kid.

As we walked into the kitchen, encountering last night's dishes and Miyako stretching out and meowing on the kitchen counter, Ken sighed.

I wanted to say I didn't understand or believe this, how could this happen, how would we get through this. But instead I asked him what we should do about dinner. "I don't care," he said, and neither did I, both of us starting to feel the weight of the phone calls ahead to our kids. So I made peanut-butter-and-jelly sandwiches that we ate quickly and thought about the scans ahead. "You think I'll be clear?" I asked Ken before we started eating.

"Absolutely," he said, both of us settling on the couch to eat in between calling our kids.

We dialed Forest first, who lived in town in a big hippie cooperative house. He had recently finished his journalism degree. It was his day off from working at the food co-op and he answered on the first ring, somewhere in the middle of a daily ten-mile walk while he listened to podcasts, spanning one edge of town to its opposite edge.

"Hey, what's up? How are you?" he asked gently without yet knowing.

"We're okay but we've been better," Ken said.

"So guess what?" I said as if this wasn't big news. "My eye was seeing things a little blurry, and it turns out I have eye cancer."

He exhaled loudly. I imagined him on the corner of a neighborhood with colorful bungalows and yard art sculptures of cats and dinosaurs. At least, that's where I hoped he was.

We explained this was a big deal, but we could treat it and I would be okay. He listened carefully, asked when the surgery would be and how long it would take to recover, if I'd lose my vision in my eye, and most of all, how I was feeling. He was a person who became totally absorbed in the present in conversations. I could feel him breathing alongside us, gauging his worry by ours which, although we tried to hide on a high shelf, he still felt.

"I can come out tonight," he said.

"It's okay," I told him.

"How are you doing?" he asked again. His gentleness made me cry just enough that it was hard to swallow the last bite of the sandwich.

We called Daniel next, in Madison, Wisconsin, where he was working on a master's in prairie restoration. His mother's son, he asked a lot of questions. He wanted to know what kind of gold, how big the tumor was, if the radiation would damage my face or brain, what stage the cancer was, if I'd be okay, and if I'd really be okay. We told him we didn't know the answers to most of his questions and also that Dr. Desai said not to research this cancer on the internet because it was too rare and not yet understood. Also, there were twenty-seven stages, but where I was in that line-up, unlike turtle names, meant very little, so don't worry about naming the stage. We said I'd be okay, repeatedly, even though we didn't know, then aimed our talk toward scans that I would surely come through with the flying colors of no abnormalities.

"What's up?" Natalie said quickly when we reached her. An aspiring electronic dance music composer and singer with a side hustle as a waitress in a Minneapolis club, she was taken completely by surprise. "You what?" We told her again. "Should I come home? I could take off work." No, we said, it's okay. "What can I do to help?"

"Pray," I said quietly. Then added in a higher voice, "but it'll be okay." She was shaken up enough that I handed Ken my phone so he could talk with her for a while, about their shared fascination with haunting Netflix series or experimental music.

I took Ken's phone and went out to the deck to call Victoria, one of my oldest friends who now lived in Wichita, where she ran with the Lebanese Orthodox. "I'll pray for you," she said, and I was grateful she would be thinking of me while gazing into the eyes of all the icons in her home and church.

I called Harriet, a good friend for many years, who appropriately cursed and commiserated with me and promised to stay in touch. She did, often texting me daily to see how I was or sending love notes. I reached out to Joy, an old pal I had lost track of for some years but happily reunited with only a few months earlier. Someone who truly embodied her name, she promised to pray for me and send chocolate (which she did).

I called Danny and Kat, whom I met at the first fabled (in my own mythology) Kansas Area Watershed Council event out in '82. They each got on an extension and listened carefully to every detail, Kat asking what kind of support I needed and Danny saying we could take one of our long walks soon, whenever I wanted.

I reached out to Suzanne, an old friend who lived in Vermont, and we talked about all we survived already in our lives. Her voice was warm as good soup, and she listened deeply to all I said. I connected with Anne, our yoga teacher and a close friend, who listened intently, then said, "Oh, shit" and "I'm totally there for you," which she was.

I called back everyone I spoke with the day before plus so many others, short but potent calls, each like manna in the desert to me. Each time we repeated the same story, one we weren't wedded to but were certainly getting serious about, conversation by conversation. At the same time, spreading out the weight of the news made us both feel a little lighter even if a lot more tired.

By 10 p.m., I was talked-out and so was Ken. We had to get up early the next morning, but first we watched an episode of the *Great British Baking Show*, one we'd seen twice before where Nadiya won. We cried with her at the end, her beautiful brown face framed by her black hijab, her beautiful brown eyes shining as she said, "I'm never going to put boundaries on myself again. I'm never going to say maybe. I'm never going to say I can't. I can and I will."

The next morning, humid already at 9 a.m., I distracted myself by thinking of a name for a new female turtle, or maybe it wasn't a distraction at all, but a way to take in the larger breathing and changing world. If it was cold enough to wear boots, I would have been shaking in them, but instead, I thought of the name Lydia, then the song, "Oh, Lydia, oh, Lydia, have you met Lydia/ Lydia, the tattooed lady" that Groucho sings from the Marx Brothers movie. Within a few days, I would name a crafty male turtle "Groucho."

Between phone calls with oncologists' offices to set up scans and tests, I named Yoda although all turtles look like Yoda. Then again, many of these turtles also look like Gandalf (the Green), which I bestowed on a very old male, surely the incarnation of the previous Gandalf.

I told myself to take heart from the turtles: they burrow underground—a process called brumation—for almost half the year, making their way back out to the air sometime each spring, blinking at the sun, feeling the air on their necks, ready to steadily crawl from one curious place to another.

2

Back in the Cancer Rodeo

There's nothing like being thrown off a bucking bronco to discover that yes, you can hit the ground hard, hobble back to your feet, and get back on, especially if you have people bringing you chicken soup and dark chocolate at regular intervals. When I was at my first cancer rodeo, I learned that helpers, just as Mr. Rogers said, would emerge from all corners.

The spring day I found out I flunked my mammogram in 2002, I was driving through the Flint Hills with Jerry and a few other friends, getting lost down a long gravel road that we thought was taking us to someone's home. Instead, it vanished in a field of tall grass thrashing itself in the big wind, under the sparkling blue sky and the sun everywhere. We did a U-turn until we found our way, but we were lost for a long time.

Being in the cancer rodeo is a lot like that. It turned out I didn't just have a little spot of breast cancer swiftly removed before I could get back to my regular programming. The cancer had spread into some lymph nodes. I also had the BRCA1 genetic mutation, which increased the risk of breast cancer exponentially along with boosting the chance of ovarian cancer, and in my father's case, the pancreatic cancer that killed him in early 2003.

There were three big surgeries, each one akin to holding onto a mechanical bull in the middle of a sandstorm. It meant surrendering to the anesthesia and waking up to soreness, nausea, and clearing skies. There were also months of chemo, mounting one unbroken pony after another with the certainty that I would be thrown off, my white cells and mojo plummeting. I'd be overtaken by a numbing white sleeve of sleep at any moment interspersed with steroid-induced closet re-organizing at 3 a.m. Ken, my family, friends, and big community love got me through. They filled our refrigerator with blintzes and chicken casseroles for the six months of chemo, drove the kids to and from piano lessons and hospital visits, brought me a TV and VCR (we had neither beforehand) so I could zone out on Steve Martin movies, and talked me through fear storms.

Breast cancer didn't prepare me for eye cancer, and all our years trying to save the land didn't prepare us for how the story would unfold. Both were like a tornado turning up in Maine or a 90-degree day in February instead of an ice storm. Furthermore, this rodeo isn't optional for most of us: we will either be formally saddled up or be helping someone else getting up from the ground. Having facilitated writing workshops for people with cancer and other serious illnesses through Turning Point, part of the KU Med Center, I've learned a few tips from the pros. For example, the time between the word "cancer" is spoken to you and a precise diagnosis and treatment plan is often the most excruciating part.

Also, cancer and treatment doesn't change who we are but rather reveals it. Big dances with mortality show us more of our essential being, and that is a priceless gift of perspective. The word "denial" is not a dirty word but a necessary coping mechanism because it's impossible to walk upright while carrying heavy rocks.

I wrote in a blog post after my diagnosis, "While I don't own a pair of red cowgirl boots, I can barely ride a horse, and I can't yodel to save my life, I can be brave enough to let all these people and procedures save my life." I didn't completely believe this yet, but words are powerful. At the same time, no one is immune to mortality, and as someone who reads the last page of any novel first, not knowing where the story goes was driving me crazy.

It also drove me to therapy, and this time with Ken. We trotted up the eighteen steps from the entrance on Massachusetts Street, the main street of Lawrence, to my therapist's office. I had brought Ken to the therapist two years earlier after he lost a job he loved for over 27 years, when we were both spinning in oil spills of anxiety.

We quickly settled on Valerie's leather loveseat. I kicked off my shoes, sat cross-legged, and placed a plush pink pillow on my lap as a makeshift desk for my journal, ready to take notes to make sense of it and to avoid feeling the full impact. Ken just crossed his legs and leaned back.

Within minutes, I got caught in a morass of questions with no answers, all beginning with "what if." What if the cancer comes back? What if my scans aren't clear? And the biggie I couldn't even say so just asked, "What if I die before I'm ready?"

Valerie didn't, at this tender session, tell me what she would say months later: Lots of us die before we're ready, which at the time catapulted us into singing the chorus to Blood, Sweat and Tears' "And When I Die..." while laughing. There was no laughing now. Instead, she talked about how GAD—my happy-sounding but very common diagnosis of Generalized Anxiety Disorder—feeds off the food of uncertainty, and the banquet table was overflowing now.

Maybe our hearts are like a set of size-descending Russian wooden dolls we keep opening until we find the solid wooden tiny one at the center. Maybe there is no solid core of us at the center but something much more mutable. "I'm just so scared," I said.

She leaned forward, her long black hair falling toward me, to show me she was serious. "There's nothing immediately to be afraid of." My fear was rooted in imagination. Also, let's reframe that 30-50% chance of metastases to a 50-70% chance no recurrence. "What the doctor was saying to you was 'You'll probably be okay, but we'll keep checking,'" she said.

The heavy clouds outside her north-facing window were building, something I knew Ken, who tracked weather like our cats track mice, was watching. Most likely it was all he could do not to pull out his phone and look at radar to determine what was coming and how fast. He didn't have questions, he said. "But how are you?" I asked him. "This must be really hard for you."

"I'm fine," he said too fast. "I'm okay. I'm really fine." We both knew he wasn't, but he was in rallying mode, responding to the morass of uncertainty and crazy-assed fear. Later he would tell me, "I just couldn't, because that's just a place you don't want to be if you don't have to." He was jarred awake in the middle of many nights though.

He didn't share until years past that he had researched the statistics Dr. Desai told me to avoid, the ones that lit up a 50% survival rate at best and led to many photos of people with disfigured faces and empty eye sockets. I thought of how, years after my first cancer, he told me that during one of the darker chemo labyrinth weeks, he didn't tell me how he went to the funeral of a colleague who died from breast cancer. It was excruciating for him to be there. "I knew it would freak you out," he said. I was and still am in awe of what he can carry on behalf of those he loves.

But on this day, as the rain began to pelt the window in a kind of Monet-like blur that matched how my right eye saw the world, Valerie had convinced me that I had been doing Olympic training for this kind of thing for years. "This is the big tournament," she said. "You might ride for the whole three minutes at the rodeo."

"But if I fall, I should avoid those hooves. That could be deadly," I answered.

"Look at the words you use. Don't say it's a deadly cancer. Say something more like, 'I have a weird little tumor in my eye. They're gonna treat it, and I'm going to be fine.' You're a writer so work with your words."

We talked about health PTSD and how second-time cancers as well as other serious illnesses arriving in multiples can hit harder because of what our bodies and psyches remember. I remembered. The Turning Point writers often said that the second or third diagnosis was worse, a cumulative effect over time. We get more delicate, not more hardened, from being scarred over. We get more vulnerable and porous as we age.

I could curl up like an armadillo in the desert when feeling threatened, but I could also open myself up again and deal with whatever comes. "Sit back and let things unfold. Don't rush things," she reminded me.

I started to cry and put down my journal, unable to write anymore. How could I just sit with this without pushing the river? A new storm showed its dramatic muscles through the windows to my right, and Valerie just watched me, nodding, then said, "Hey, you are the Indiana Jones of this struggle. Do you have any idea how strong you are?"

Ken and I walked down the stairs more slowly than we ran up them, hand in hand. I looked at him as he pushed open the heavy glass door to the rainy street, and he smiled broadly but his eyes were tracking the storm. The phone in my purse rang, and it was my mother, so I gave her a cheery update on our way to Limestone, the best stone oven pizza in the galaxy. I laughed with her about how she had this pizza last time she was here, and wasn't it great? Also, I would be okay, really fine, I was sure of it. I spoke with a lightness the warm rain encouraged.

With my hand on the door handle to Limestone, I heard my name and within moments, I was wrapped in the arms of Dr. Soule. Although I had an appointment with her in a few days and we had talked on the phone a few breathless (for me) and calm (for her) times, it felt like oncology homecoming week to see her.

"I'm going to be okay. I was just telling my mother that," I said. Then to my surprise, I started crying.

"Of course you're going to be okay," she said, while hugging me back.

"Okay" is a jaunty word, one that bobs on the water of waiting for scans, test results, then a semblance of life snapping back into a familiar pattern. I woke up the next day with a wide ocean of sadness, fatigue, and numbness, but I also had three turtles, two females and a male, to name.

I could see their ornate shells in the photos Ben sent, one's shell a mosaic of tiles in green, brown, and even with flecks of gold or orange. Given the biblical proportion of my sadness, I went with Leah, Jacob and Rachel from the Old Testament. Leah, whom Jacob had to marry to get to his much-desired Rachel, got a bad deal, so why not let her be a vibrant turtle of intricate patterns?

Maybe this was a rodeo with turtles instead of horses and very expensive scanning devices instead of mechanical bulls. Maybe, definitely, it wasn't a rodeo at all or anything easy to fit into the enclosure of a metaphor, but it was where I needed to live right now.

The days to come were full of scheduling scans and tests, talking myself down from the anxiety tree with friends, cleaning the floor for no good reason, listening to the soundtrack of *The Sound of Music* while typing notes to coaching clients, and planning writing workshops as if nothing was amiss. I also aimed myself toward another of my helpers:

Ursula, an energy healer I had worked closely with during breast cancer.

Back in the day of Cancer #1, she went with me to all my chemo appointments. She would hold the red bag of toxic chemicals between her steady hands and breathe healing energy into them before the nurses set up the drip into a port in my clavicle. She also came to all three of my surgeries—and for two of them, she was even allowed to be in the surgery room, all gowned up with my plastic-glove-covered hands holding the top of my head, even when my breasts were cut off my body.

How to describe what she does is like explaining the ocean to a seashell. She works with energy and color, sound and meditation. She listens closely to what the body needs and aligns it with its innate healing ability. When Ursula worked on me, I could feel shivers across my back. I was sure her hands were holding my shoulders when she wasn't even in the room. I could see wide expanses of hills, hear birds and crickets, sense that there were others in the room with us. I also needed so little pain relief after each surgery that my doctors were astonished.

Ursula is a German woman 15 years my senior. We had joked about how she was helping heal a Jew who was only alive because my grandmother got out of Poland a generation before the Holocaust. Actually, the plot deepens because Ursula was born in March of 1945 in Poland, where her family was forced after the German army took over land where her father, a forest ranger and engineer, worked. As the Russians advanced toward Poznan, her parents piled their four children, including newborn Ursula, in a horse wagon, which they pulled themselves through the woods to get the last train out of Poland. Somehow, love and livelihood brought Ursula to my hometown of Lawrence, Kansas, for a few decades and across my path.

Although Ursula was now living in her home country near the Alps, she would work with me from a distance through this cancer of the eye. We talked regularly on an app that allowed her to show me her apartment and the view of the snow-covered mountains and allowed me to share the wind-battered prairie and first blooming purple-and-white irises. It was a relief to see her familiar face framed by white hair, not quite a pageboy because of its waves, and always her brilliant blue eyes.

Even now, on a quiet Sunday morning, late afternoon where it was balmy in Kansas and crisply cold out her window, she led me in a slow breathing exercise, during which I envisioned, at her suggestions, gold and purple light running through my body. I sat on my porch, eyes closed, the phone on my lap, and let the sweat slowly run down my face in the sudden heat of a May day. Or was it tears? We would prepare, she reminded me, just like we did last time.

When I opened my eyes, I saw her looking at me from thousands of miles away. "Write your intentions," she said. Mostly my intention was to live, but I knew from experience how much it could help to write more of the details of getting from this existential threat to where the air felt sweeter, the world more generous.

"You know how to do this," Ursula said, and it struck me that Valerie had said the same thing. "Call it an eye journey, a health passage," she said, which we also agreed would be good to tell our kids.

After we said goodbye, I looked up to see my friends Julie and Vaughn parking their car and carrying a large box toward me. A few days earlier, Vaughn, a cowboy-hat-wearing western Kansas man, had told Julie in his beautiful bass voice, "If she needs red cowgirl boots, then red cowgirl boots she shall have."

Vaughn handed me the box, and I quickly slipped my bare feet into the boots, even though I was wearing shorts and a t-shirt. Standing next to Shay, I was startled by how comfortable and broken in they felt, all of us laughing at how I was now equipped to kick cancer's ass. Both Vaughn and Julie had both been through their own trials and rodeos, near-misses and impossible survivals, so they understood.

Whether this is a rodeo or a redux, I was surrounded by good people with the best senses of humor and get-up-and-go gumption because of close encounters with the life force. These are the best people you'll ever meet or even be.

3

Playlist for a PET Scan in the Cold Desert Night

"You're growing a magic eye," Laura, a storyteller (professionally as well as just who she is), told me in the tender and terrifying weeks between diagnosis and the first surgery.

In many fairy tales, she explained, the seeker is called or even forced (think Jonah and the whale) to go on an adventure—dangerous, bad-weathered, and treacherous—to save himself or her beloved or even their whole world. We must endure terrible trials, accomplish unlikely feats, and soothe the agitated monkeys of fear for an undetermined time in unknown territory. In other words, as Robert Frost once wrote, "the only way out is through."

While I don't see cancer ordeals as heroic despite clichéd notions about survivors, I do believe we can courage up to whatever life lessons we're enrolled in, despite not remembering signing up for such lessons. As many know, it's not always the big things that get us, or truly they do get us but we expect them to throw us to the ground. Like Robert Eliot says, "Rule number one is, don't sweat the small stuff. Rule number two is, it's all small stuff."

Scans can be ho-hum medical blips for some, but for those of us with lifetime memberships in Camp Claustrophobia, not so much. Between my first cancer, pancreatic cancer risk, and BRCA1-positive status, I knew what it was to be felt up by giant machines with invisible hands. I felt the terror of the metal hands gliding me into tight spaces where I was surrounded by clanging, metal-on-metal surges. I was both scared of the machines and what the machines might discover.

Sometimes fear lands us into a freezing desert in the dark, and such was true for my PET scan. On a late May morning when the temperature had unexpectedly dropped to near-freezing, the scan turned out to be one of the most terrifying events of my life. This feels ridiculous to write years later, but I can barely remember anything else that scared me quite as much, although surely, what I experienced is rooted in old trauma.

"Trauma is not what happens to you, it's what happens inside you as a result of what happened to you," says Gabor Mate, an expert on the subject and a Holocaust survivor. While I can't say where my fear of being trapped in tight spaces came from, I can remember growing up with a sense of danger closing in on me, no escape, and no power to change what was happening. My father slapped, kicked, and pushed us, and when he was really angry, bit his tongue while taking off his belt to beat my siblings and me. I understood in a very visceral way what it means to be powerless.

After my parents' divorce, I became an accidental daughter-wife for my dad, and at the same time I lost most contact with the rest of my family. My father commuted home late from the city. He demanded a perfectly-broiled steak and some vegetables not cooked into oblivion. I was too depressed to deliver the goods, and his quick agitation turned to insults, bitter sarcasm, and kicking me to the linoleum floor. Our suburban neighbors, after my mother and siblings moved out, stopped speaking to us, so biking around my block was lonely. No one so much as waved hello or nodded that yes, they did see me grow up here. Within a year, a step-family joined the mix and things got worse. I was 15, I was 16, I was 17, and perpetually on the outside looking in.

"I'm just very insecure," I would tell Phil, my high school synagogue advisor. He worked a day job as a guidance counselor in a New York City school for broken, angry, and hurt girls.

"For good reason," he replied as we sat in the hall, our backs against the painted cinderblock walls leading to Hebrew school classrooms. He listened, encouraged my writing, and affirmed that I wasn't crazy, just in a bad situation. He and a few other saving graces—an English teacher who held an after-school poetry club for what she called, she told me years later, the broken girls—gave me safe perches until I was old enough to fly on my own.

Of course, one of the sturdiest perches was poetry. I wrote about the changeable sky that never failed to entertain and the beautiful world, cherry blossoms and all, unfolding around me even if I felt alone. I was always a curious kid, and I told myself then that if I could just hold on, things would get more interesting, likely even better.

It's no wonder that decades later, my mother-in-law, Alice, and I swapped stories of how we stood up to or escaped our fathers' beatings, giving us the strength to make a much more peaceable life. We also talked about how much we loved listening to birds, watching sunsets, looking out on the newly-fallen snow when the living room was dark except for Christmas lights. We understood that no matter what happened in our lives, our childhoods would always remain the hardest thing. This is still true for me.

Yet something of the old agony remains in many of us. Sudden sounds make me jump as well as when someone comes up to me from behind. My close friends know if they get to the table in the restaurant first, they should save the seat against the wall for me. The dogs of hyper-vigilance are lean and muscular in my psyche from regular runs.

So what does this have to do with getting a PET scan forty years later? I don't have a Venn diagram to show the overlap, only that there's spark-to-spark connection between being alone, beaten, and ostracized as a teen and lying on a metal table sliding in and out of a humming machine decades later. Something lingered despite all the therapy, Rolfing, energy healing, writing, and season after season, year after year, of big love from family, friends, and community. Trauma is a spiked animal, easily startled when interrupted from its long hibernation.

The night before and morning of the PET scan, I was antsy, unable to talk with Ken without arguing with him for having the nerve to ask me things like if I wanted any water while we waited. He was in a similar state, picking a fight with me as we drove to the hospital because we left ten minutes late. We both had our pointy flares out and were taking no prisoners.

When we got to the hospital, an older woman—I'll call her Betty, who was a volunteer, angel, or both—escorted us through the entire hospital from the east to the west side, then outside to an RV-like vehicle, not for conventional trips. It was a PET scan on wheels that parked at one medical center before taking thousands of dollars of high-tech equipment down the road to the next hospital.

We had to ride up an open metal elevator ramp to the entrance. Once inside, I saw the machine, a long table that went in and out of a large, white plastic donut. At first, I wasn't too scared until I found out there was no bathroom in the vehicle. Nikki, the tech, gave me an injection of a sugar solution with a slightly radiative substance that worked as a tracer for the scan. With her high forehead, large blue eyes, and pointy chin, she looked a little like an anime character but with none of the charm. When I told her I was claustrophobic, so please be patient with me, she rolled her eyes and said she was on a tight schedule. I took a Lorazepam to relax and practiced breathing slowly in and out for counts of four, instantly knowing I had to pee right away by virtue of there being no place to go.

Ken explained, while Nikki injected the sugar solution, how PET scan works: "The sugar is absorbed faster in tumors than in other living tissue. The radioactive particles degrade into matter and anti-matter (electrons and positrons), and the sensors pick up the positrons to pinpoint the location of any tumors." So basically, I was being infused with anti-matter. Nikki nodded that this was more or less true.

We went back to the main hospital to wait for an hour for the tracer to circulate through my body, parking ourselves on a long crescent-shaped couch, built into a curve of wall near the gift shop that specialized in sunflower-covered journals, small stuffed giraffes, and crystal angels. I passed the time reading about South American bluebirds in an old *National Geographic* and checking Facebook every five minutes on my phone. I also watched a video three times of a man playing trombone to lure cows cross a field.

Eventually Betty, who favored purple silk tops and multiple, purple-beaded necklaces, came to escort me to the scan. Because the RV was so small, Ken couldn't be there at all, and on this blustery day, he went to wait in his small Honda.

When I first lay down on the table, Nikki tried to strap a kind of plastic straight jacket around me to keep my arms still. As my blood pressure shot up, I told her there was no way I was going to wear that, and I promised to keep my hands tucked under my hips and not move my arms. I also found out that I couldn't wear my earbuds with my special music, a playlist I put together just for the occasion, but we got my laptop set up to play my PET scan soundtrack. My heart was off to the races, and we hadn't even begun.

As Nikki moved me into position to have the machine measure me, panic grew exponentially until I called out to her to come give me a second Lorazepam. I was fighting with all I had to stay put, even as my neurotic angels were banging the drum for me to leave immediately. Nikki brought me a second pill from my purse, and she said I needed to stay very still. There were other people after me. I was crazy thirsty, and she said she couldn't bring me any more water except for the sip to swallow the pill.

She went back to the control room to continue the scan, and big-teethed fear gripped my thoughts. My whole torso trembled, my fingers and toes got cold, and my breath shortened. But then the music began. I took a slower breath, trying to keep my shaking from screwing up the scan and landing me back to do it all again next week.

The music helped as Brandi Carlile's this-is-truth-voice began singing "The Joke" about how those of us living brave lives will eventually triumph. In the chorus, she belts out, "I have been to the movies, and I know the way the story ends," telling those of us who feel beaten down by the status quo that we have the strength and bravery to make a happy ending.

I sensed Ursula was in the room with me. That might be possible considering that numerous times before, when she was actually in the room with me working on my head. I still felt her hands holding my feet. I realized I was surrounded by help, whether wrought by my imagination or gifted from beyond my little brain.

But none of this calmed me. My heart raced, I was breathing so hard that I was making my throat sore, and I wanted with all my might to run, even if I had to navigate an elevator ramp to do it. *Calm down,* I told myself with my in-breath. *I can't,* I answered myself with my out-breath.

Yet, yet: I had to give myself over to whatever it was for however long to make sure the cancer was contained. Only then could I begin the treatment that would save my life. That *could* save my life.

I was still freaking out when Vaughn Williams's "Fantasia on Greensleeves," that classical variation on a folk song, came on. I saw an imaginary Ursula standing at my head, her steady hands holding the base of my skull. I let the weight of my head sink into her hands as the machine read my torso.

After a while, I realized I was in a desert at night—it was cold (the room I was in was freezing), and I was parched and so thirsty, there alone with a little pup tent I had set up. I stood on the dry ground and looked at the stars. I felt so scared and so much in awe at all the beauty at once. The depth and crowded light of that night sky made me feel like I was falling upward just like all those times I saw dark night skies in unpopulated swaths of western Kansas or at high altitudes in rural Colorado when the air was so cold that nothing warmed me, but those stars!

Ellis Delaney's "How Would It Be" started. "What if all of our mistakes are forgiven?" What would that mean for the house of the story where I lived? I remembered the kid I was, the teen I turned into. I believed, as children are prone to, that my suffering and abuse were my own fault. What if my mistakes weren't all my own? I looked at the ground, lit in billions of specks of light, slivers of what's above, between bundles of hedgehog cacti and desert sage.

Broken open in relief and also wondering at the cool air on my skin and the stars sharpening in the dark, I could see more of the swath of the Milky Way. I could be here, out in the open, the little tent behind me, the edgy brush visible in the starlight as I waited. Maybe a vole was moving through the grasses in the distance, maybe a mule deer.

Greg Greenway was singing "I Carry Your Heart in Me," a song based on e.e. cummings' poem of the same title. I breathed in the lyrics, "The secret that nobody knows, from root to bud of the tree that knows, higher than the soul can hold, is you." I lay down on the bare ground, a little lumpy and cold, avoiding anything prickly, and closed my eyes. My rushing heart slowed. Someone's hand was on my chest, right in the center, breathing warmth into me. . . .

I opened my eyes, the room dimly lit and buzz-humming to its machine self. I closed my eyes, and I was back in the desert, alone and not alone. The old imaginary friends I had forgotten about from my childhood were right here—Monday, Tuesday, Wednesday, Thursday, and all the others—each of them created to make up for my lack of real friends. I was four or five when they came into my life, accompanying me daily, each on their day of the week.

Then they were gone, but the air felt less wind-driven. *It's okay,* I told myself, and I finally believed it. Mary Chapin Carpenter's "Jericho" further spoke to befriending the darkness within, starting with "You can't see me yet/ Seeing takes a long, long time." Freezing on the desert floor at that moment, I knew this long time would take the rest of my life. I also felt at peace, even though I was so thirsty and alone in the desert. The song is named "Jericho" because of the biblical story about Joshua blowing his horn and making the walls of the city come tumbling down. The song tells us, "We are all the places that we've been." What was falling down?

Decades ago, when Ursula was working on me as I lay on her massage table, bird song abounded and penetrated the windows. I felt, saw, even tasted dying and death. It seemed utterly thrilling, a night sky launched with stars and space, motion and love, love, love. "But I choose life, I choose long life," I told the moment. Whatever and however death happens, it will be so different than anything I can imagine, so outlandishly expansive and beyond who I am, that there's nothing to be afraid of, I knew then.

I knew this in the PET scan room too. Then the lights came on. Nikki and Betty entered the room to turn me around so that I would go feet-first into the machine. Dolly Parton's "Here You Go Again" came on. Betty and I talked about how much we loved Dolly and this song, and how Betty is very claustrophobic too. Nikki told me to hold my hands together at the center of my chest and continue to wear my eye pad. The machine took me into itself again. Halfway done.

Music continued its narrative. Carrie Newcomer sang, "The empty space has changed somehow/ And it's filled with hallelujah now," from her song "Arrival." I felt hallelujah all over me. I sensed Ursula's hands on my feet. But there was someone else too: I realized Betty was back in the room, and about four or five times, she squeezed my left arm supportively. I wanted to thank her, but I was trying to stay still for the end of the scan.

Then it was over.

I asked Nikki where Betty was because I wanted to thank her for holding my arm. She said no one was in the room. But actually, it felt like a cast of thousands.

I left the RV, taking a strand of stairs down to Ken, who was waiting in the nearby car. When I got in, I started crying too hard to talk. "What happened?" he asked.

"Everything," I said between gulps of crying. "It was cold," I said. "I was in the desert." I blew my nose and exhaled quickly. "The desert," I told him. "The stars. . . . Jericho too."

"What do you want now?" he asked, his hand on my shoulder as he tilted toward me. I pulled out all the tissues I could find from my purse, some crumpled up but still serviceable.

Finally, I got myself steadied down to just ebbing hard breaths and tears. "I want," I tried to say, then had to make another run at it, "I want French toast."

He backed out the car, and we headed to Wheatfields, a bakery in town where we soon made it a tradition that after every scan, for years to come, we'd come here for the crisp bacon, sometimes the almond croissant, always the hot tea, all the food returning me to where I never left. Grounding me.

That night as I was standing on the back deck, looking at the dark landscape of this much more humid place than the desert, soon to be filled with lightning bugs and other wonders of the dark, I got a text from Ben. He found a turtle who had survived a long time and kept growing in pattern and vibrancy. She was old, beautiful, and vibrant. I had named her Ursula.

4

Herculia the Turtle

We named her Herculia because she needed a strong name, Ben and I agreed as he stood on our porch and carefully, with a pair of tweezers, removed some of the botflies that destroyed her back legs. He had just found her upside down in a just-burned prairie in the county and stopped at our house to borrow some tweezers. We had both looked at her charred shell, some of its top layer flaking off, right before I rummaged through the medical cabinet for a pair of tweezers to remove botflies, a type of parasite.

"She's probably not going to make it," he told me. "But I'll try everything I can," he added, looking up from under his long brown bangs that covered his eyelids.

"But if you get out all the botflies, won't she be fine?"

"Her back legs will still be so damaged that she won't be able to get around."

He took her to his lab, where she became a mascot for the Washburn biology department, everyone cheering her on. But she still wouldn't eat. The department secretary took Herculia outside every day, placed her in the grass to soak up being directly on the earth although she couldn't propel herself forward yet. Six weeks later, she finally ate a small worm, so maybe she would make it after all. We already planned how Ken—who customized wheelchairs as an occupational therapist—and Ben would make a wheelchair prosthesis, a kind of miniature wheelbarrow, for her back legs. We imagined her pulling herself across the warm green grass of campus.

My own medical conveyer belt continued clicking along until we could turn toward the surgery room. Next station: a closed MRI to make sure there was no brain tumor in the mix. This would require claustrophobia mitigation in the form of medication to knock me out. Just a week earlier, I was in Dr. Soule's office, hearing the results of the PET scan: all clear. She held my hand when she said this, then reassured me that the meds would make the MRI much easier than the PET scan.

In the prep room for the MRI, right before they started the drip of fentanyl and Versed—the two-drug combo that would sweep me out to sea while my head and shoulders slid into the clanging body of the MRI machine—I panicked. I tried to slow my breath, counting to four on each inhalation and exhalation, but my heart was roaring down the highway. My usual coping mechanism of getting up to pee every ten minutes was not helping. Pacing calmed me only enough not to bolt. I stared longingly at the heavy metal door from the edge of the table where I sat in my hospital gown on top, jeans, underwear, and socks on my bottom half.

"I can't do this," I told Ken after the nurse checked on me and said the radiologist would be in to meet me in a moment.

He moved his chair closer to me, took my hand, "Of course you can." He was tired from his job and a late night on the phone with Daniel, who was struggling to finish his master's thesis on prairie restoration and arguing with every suggestion Ken offered. I noticed Ken's hair was looking more gray than brown all of sudden.

"Why can't they start the drugs right now?" Like so many things in Cancerland, it's the waiting that gets you.

The door burst open, and a balding man with very shiny silver tufts of hair over his considerable ears, walked in. So did Kate, a small white woman with a buzz cut, purple scrubs, and elaborate floral tattoos vining up her arms. He was carrying a chart but not smiling. "So you have some claustrophobia," he said. "The drugs should help but not always." I looked past him toward the door. I could stand, politely say, "Excuse me," then make a run for the car, but I should remember then to take my purse so that I'd have the keys.

"It's very narrow in there. Some people do okay. Some people don't," he added as if he were sent by the devil to fluff up the cotton candy of fear expanding in my stomach. "Yes, that is a rather tight MRI machine." I don't know what, if anything else, he said next because my mind was so busy with fight-or-flight mechanics, each step from here to home being plotted at triple-speed.

When he was gone, Kate rushed over and told me not to worry, it would be fine, and she reached out her hand to hold mine. I noticed that among the roses and violets, she had a lapis heart tattooed on her right tricep. "That's beautiful," I told her.

"Thanks," she said. "It's for my grandmother. She was a cool lady."

"Did she grow flowers too?"

Kate laughed while grasping my forearm. "Nah, that's me. I'm just crazy for flowers."

Then we were walking to the room which, magically enough, was lit in turquoise, lapis, and purple lights, all of my favorite colors, making the space into a Bollywood movie spa.

"I love these colors," I told her.

"Yeah, a lot of people do," she answered.

One of the technicians, a slight man with ample black beard and happy blue eyes, leaned over me to say, "We can change the colors to whatever you want."

"No, this is great," I said, although I wouldn't move from my perch on the table to lying down until they asked me several times. It turned out Kate could hold my right hand, Ken could hold my left, and I could listen to any music I wanted as they started the drip of drugs, a quick stairway into oblivion. I chose Enya, having learned long ago how her music was perfectly balanced to fill in the small quiet spaces between the banging teeth and booming echoes of the machine.

I lay down, telling myself to breathe, while Enya sang "Orinoco Flow." It turned out there was a quiet pond at the top of my head, a lot of space around it with no trees for miles, fog rolling in, a small bird singing in the voice of an Irish New Age singer. I felt Kate's warm hand. The turquoise and purple lights told me it was going to be okay, with bigger space opening between some old fear that I could be buried alive and the countering logic that it was just a machine I was visiting for an astonishingly small percentage of my days.

The pond had an old rusting chair nearby, something that was once turquoise but still smooth, decades old. I sat there and discovered it rocked just a little in time with the water. Glints of light wove themselves along the surface of water, then vanished under the next ripple. I reached down and picked up a smooth, flat black stone, rounded with white speckles. I remembered finding this at the Oregon coast a few years ago, and how it reminded me of Jerry. A decade before I visited this very beach, he was there, afterwards telling me all about and showing me his photographs of rocks balancing against orange and blue sky.

Then I thought of how he died, after being alone in his apartment from a very aggressive virus long before COVID. We wouldn't know why he didn't call any of us for help until after we scattered his ashes across the Akin's Prairie in our county. It turned out he had an aneurysm in his neck that was impinging on his memory, so much so that he missed his doctor's appointment to get it fixed. We couldn't put the story together until after we—his brothers and sisters from mostly Minnesota and his friends from Kansas—shook those light ashes out of the plastic baggie to let the wind sweep them across reddening grasses or our jeans.

It is so often like this: we think we see the whole sky, but really, it's just a sliver of light or cloud cover. We think we see the prairie grasses, but what's above ground is less than a half of the underground roots. Even this MRI could only reveal a glimmer of what was and what wasn't.

I was quickly teleported back to Spa Bollywood, where Kate was helping me sit up, people all around saying, "You were great" as if I just performed an aria to a sold-out crowd.

As we pulled into our parking spot off our long gravel driveway, there were suddenly dozens of hackberry butterflies, even though this wasn't their usual time. One landed on the end of my finger as I pointed at the butterflies. Ken and I both looked at her as she opened her closed wings and vanished into the cedars. "That was weird," he said. I nodded.

"Is this harder?" I asked him as we walked up the steps and opened the front door. We were making our way onto the porch to plop down. He preferred the old futon propped up on one side by two bricks and a hardback-covered dictionary from the 1960s. He didn't answer at first, something as common for him as stopping in the middle of a sentence to go feed the dog while I tapped my foot impatiently in one of those New-Yorker-married-to-a-Kansan moments. "And don't just say, 'I don't know.'"

Ken smiled a little and turned to me. "It's different. It was a lot clearer last time, and we could research just about anything about breast cancer. But this," he paused as we listened to what sounded like a car, then he got up to see and I followed. A military helicopter was passing over, just skirting the northwest sky above the farm.

"What the fuck?" Ken said, which I repeated, but I was thinking of something else. There would be quarterly scans, Dr. Desai had recently told us, for at least ten years, then continued scans but not so often. It was hard to fathom how long we'd have to be on the watch. How, with this cancer, the usual anniversaries of survival didn't apply. Then again, such anniversaries are arbitrary since our bodies swirl with cancer cells most of the time and won't do damage. When it comes to the big potentials—life and death and all the heartaches, struggles, and unknowns in between—it's often impossible to point to an exact origin point.

Ken shook his head until the helicopter was out of sight, then we returned to the porch, me in my favorite seat, a comfortable but hideous chartreuse plush chair Daniel got from a thrift store for college years ago. I took three extra-strength Tylenol, more than the recommended allotment, guzzled iced tea, then picked up the conversation again. "So how is it different?"

"This one just came out of left field. There's no assurance that something big isn't around the corner," he said, but then he got a text he wanted to answer, and by the time he finished that, he fell asleep, mouth open, eyes closed.

I opened my laptop while wondering whether it made any difference that this was happening in my right eye rather than my left. I understood that the right side of the brain is the center of creativity, the vulnerable and magical part that can spot possibilities hiding in plain sight, but I always felt unfettered, bounding about like a herd of gazelles in my left-right sites of creativity. Yet there was also the loss of control, and it doesn't take a control freak to understand the metaphor here. It wasn't just Dr. Desai who said not to look up ocular melanomas on the internet because it's both a rare and deadly cancer with limited research on treatment effectiveness. Dr. Soule said the same thing. And Valerie. And Dr. Sandal. And Ursula. Don't try to find answers so you can have the illusion of control. Just acknowledge this moment of fuzzy vision and clear-seeing, chaos and balance, beauty and pain.

I closed the laptop, put it on the table beside me, and loving the warm breeze, opted to quietly step out of the porch to the side yard. Looking up into the Osage orange tree, I thought of how I saw myself over the years. When I was a teenager and young adult, I saw myself as a victim, wishing upon star after star for some tether to a family and community, some semblance of being loved without having to prove myself. I narrated my story as if it were a screenplay because it was too hard to acknowledge that I had swallowed the poison of believing I was a failure, a screw-up, a selfish girl.

But I learned to make peppermint tea and cinnamon scones out of low self-esteem and gumption, crafting a life out of all that had saved me as a kid: poetry, a sense of God in the trees, and a hunger to do something that made a difference.

I also wanted most of all to be loved, and lo and behold, I found Ken, this man snoring beside me, having repositioned himself to sleep on his side folded up as best he could on the too-short futon couch. First we were friends, comrades-in-arms in our small bioregional group. We met often at potlucks where everyone brought carob brownies or tabouli before we made newsletters out of typed pages, rubber cement, and press-on lettering.

A year after meeting, Ken and I were naked in his bed late at night because we were tired and we were at an age and in a community where people slept nude in a non-sexual way without thinking any-thing of it. But something else overtook us. I told myself this was a proximity thing, that he would soon reject me for greener pastures, something previous boyfriends had taught me. For five years, every so often, I thought so loudly, "But you're going to leave me soon, right?" that I accidentally said it. He tilted his head like dogs when hearing an indiscernible-to-humans whistle and answer, "What the fuck are you talking about?"

Meanwhile, real friends became family while I rebuilt my relation-ship with my family of origin. I found additional family in Ken's parents and sisters, then Ken and I made our family together. Conception to birth to Legos on the floor, stuffed kitty cats in the bed, and live tree frogs in the tank. So much has saved me, but finally, life isn't a safe bet.

I recalled: the agony of almost losing Daniel at birth when he swallowed amniotic fluid and wouldn't come to for minutes. The terror of almost losing Forest in a terrible accident when I hit a patch of black ice while driving all the kids to school in the minivan that plummeted into a ravine. I had to remember all the healing and relief I was blessed beyond blessed to receive despite the slippery slope of deaths too overwhelming to bear.

Even breast cancer—with its hot and cold walks through chemo and surgeries, sleeping off anesthesia, and eating the cheesy chicken casserole someone left—hadn't felt existentially threatening for more than handfuls of minutes. Even when the news opened its jaws and told me how iffy the years ahead might be, people filled my mailbox, inbox, and refrigerator with love. The kids, Ken, my friends, my family wrapped tight around me to say *no matter what* and *it's okay*.

What story had I been telling myself about being too intense or too much or not enough? What lens was I looking through to see this beautiful world? Was I a recovering self-savior, a fix-it bee warrior, a competence junkie, a lost child, a recovering under-achiever? Was I running from my own fear all these years? Was I blind to what I was actually living?

I remembered something Kim Stafford, a wonderful poet from Oregon, told me about his mother's prescription for a good life: "An hour of beauty a day." Here I was each day, almost always on the porch, listening. Amidst bird song or fights—it was hard to tell or know which winged being was involved. A large truck on the highway half a mile away. A plane overhead, aiming west. The wind gathering itself, then surging. I opened my eyes and saw what looked like an oak leaf tilting one side, then another on its slow way down to the litter.

"Live in the layers/ not in the litter," Stanley Kunitz wrote in "The Layers," one of my favorite poems. But he also wrote that, although he couldn't yet decipher it, "no doubt the next chapter/ in my book of transformations/ Is already written./ I am not done with my changes." The layers spun out horizontally through these emerging woods: the new trails Ken and Daniel were macheting into being through the cedars. Even the invasive honeysuckle Ken weeded, cut, and burned regularly. Everything—what helps, what harms—everywhere, they teach how we're just another thing among things.

At the same time, all these things were getting even more indistinct. My 2004 mud-splashed Honda CRV parked nearby, the telephone pole, and a loud bird swooping low and up and again were hard to distinguish from each other except for shadows trembling more. The phone startled me. The MRI showed my head was unfettered by cancer even if it was lost in its own searchlights of fear, especially since the vision in my right eye was noticeably declining.

When Ken and I went back to see Dr. Desai, I was sure the tumor must be growing quickly. Was it too late to stop this train? Within an hour of arrival, we were greatly relieved to discover that my eyesight was being impinged instead by fluid build-up in my eye, which was of course made worse by stress. After Dr. Desai gave us this news, we were sent to meet the radiation oncologist, a Dr. Patel, in another wing of the hospital.

Getting to his office in the far-off freezing hinterlands of the medical center turned out to be a maze that would thwart test rats. The lights along the way glared garish fluorescence down sanatorium-gray halls, so empty and vast they seemed as uninhabited as the moon. I finally found a desk and a person behind a window. Then we were in an examining room, just a chair, a table, and a counter under twitching fluorescence.

Dr. Patel was from Mumbai, and like my adopted nieces, spoke softly and calmly. His brown eyes held steady as he answered our questions. Likely no nausea. Perhaps some headaches. This implant option, he let us know, was so much more effective and less damaging than having radiative waves shot into my eye repeatedly for days. What to do for the five days I'm positively glowing? Rest, just rest.

He explained I would either go home for those five days, needing to keep a distance away from humans and animals, or, if the radiation level was too high, stay in the hospital. My stomach tightened so I started pleading my case. I'm an earth girl who needs to be outside every day in the air and especially wind if I'm to heal. "Don't fence me in," I might have belted out while explaining that a sterile and remote hospital room, likely in which the windows wouldn't even open, would be devastating for me. And my bed, please, can I sleep in my own bed?

"We just have to see what your radiation levels are. It's a very objective decision," he told me with great patience, nodding to show me that he got it about why I wanted to go home.

On the way home, I thought of the turtles. It doesn't take a rocket scientist or a turtle biologist to see the parallels between messy humans and these ancient and resilient beings, although I'm sure the turtles outrun us in patience and grace. How could they hibernate so long each year, and emerge into the mud, rain, and wind of messy and changeable spring, finding their footing through storms and droughts, trials and tenderness?

Turtles pre-date humans, their ancestor proto-turtles as much as 220 million years old. Ben explained to me the last time I saw him, "Many species are virtually unchanged morphologically since the dinosaurs, which is pretty incredible."

Incredible indeed, and so is simply holding a turtle, marveling at her ability to live below and among us, navigating water and land, earth and fire with a hard shell that tells her stories of age and art, and inside that shell, a beating heart is committed to life. According to Hindu mythology, our world rests on the back of a turtle, who rests on the back of another and another, turtles all the way down, much like our own healing journeys. So let me pause and name what gives us strength and sight, and remember just how mortal we are.

As Ben texted me daily reports on Herculia, it sure sounded like she was going to make it. She was eating more, and she tried to pull herself forward with her front claws, making slow inroads into mobility again. She would persist, this wounded, left-for-dead turtle, for a few months.

But later in the summer, after my surgeries, Ben would meet me on the front porch to tell me Herculia had died, and we would both cry.

5
Tornado

The humidity was insufferable so I turned the air-conditioning to "high" in the hot car, windows open to wave out the old air, as I drove out to the Pendleton farm for peonies on Memorial Day because I love peonies and the Pendletons. Karen and John, grade school friends of Ken's, were famous for their asparagus as well as their corn maze, one year shaped like a bee by field art artist Stan Herd. But they're also peony whisperers, and as a woman who loves the scent of those wild balls of blossom, I had to get a bundle of them.

I arrived at closing time, none of us knowing that my sale would be the last for months, after destruction required unburying wooden slats and bulldozing what couldn't be lifted by human hands. I saw John as soon as I circled the market building where dozens of peonies waited patiently in refrigerated buckets. Although I was there for the flowers, why not get some new plants for the garden? Soon we were threading through the greenhouse, talking tomatoes, talking peppers, talking about how growing vegetables and flowers was financially marginal and physically exhausting.

This led us to weather. In 2006, a March microburst—a powerful downdraft that plummets from sky to ground, sometimes causing as much damage as a good-sized tornado—powered down on the farm, damaging every building and just about every piece of farm equipment. It came so quickly that John ended up diving underneath a desk to wait it out, telling our local paper, "It sounded like a dozen 747s sitting on top of the building going full bore."

When I told him how amazing it was that they rebuilt and persevered, especially given that the microburst was not their first big weather experience, he said, "You know, I tell myself that if something like that happens again, it's time to just throw in the towel. It's too much." It was unusually hot, and we were both sweating in the intoxicating scent of a thousand tomato plants begging me to adopt them all. "The hours, the work, it's a lot. You'd think I could just retire someday like a normal person."

"But none of us are normal people," I said, and we both laughed. I walked toward Karen, who fetched those heavy balls on the ends of long stems while talking about the care and feeding of them. "Just plop them in a vase, and magic!" she said, then asked me for an eye update. I bought a dozen white, pink, and fuchsia peonies. They hold tight in the womb stage of flowerhood, then pop open, big as faces, holding nothing back. Within a week, they start dropping petals and fall apart. "If you were a flower," a friend told me years ago, "you'd be a peony."

I took offense at the time, wanting to will myself into the delicate willowy curves of the iris or perhaps a flashy red-and-white striped rose that requires a hothouse and regular pruning. But my friend was right: I'm a thrasher against reality, a tight wrap around what I think until I'm irritated enough that I explode out of it, even if it exhausts me in the process.

The next day I watched the Pendletons' peonies unfurl into full-throttle fireworks of blossoms. The heft and heat of the air made me feel like I was going to lose my mind, yet I was surprised by how little it took to bring the blossoms out of seclusion, just a vase, some cool water, and a night. With this cancer scare, I knew the bold and brave peony was what I needed on my night table.

By late afternoon, the air was so weighted in humidity that it was hard to think straight or breathe freely. Kris said to me on the phone that if anything ever felt like tornado weather, this was it. Daniel had called earlier in the day to say he was reading radar, and it looked like something could happen here. I told Kris it was just fucking weird, and surely nothing really happens all that tornadic here, but maybe there would be hail and high winds, our usual outcome from frightening forecasts.

Then I got into my car to pick up a rotisserie chicken from the grocery store, maybe some salad too because it was too hot to cook. But as I turned right on 31st Street to head to the store, I noticed the greenish black horizon in the rear-view mirror. Laura Lorson, one of my favorite voices on Kansas Public Radio, told us there was a significant weather event coming to our area. "If you can hear my voice, you are in a tornado watch and thunderstorm warning," she said.

A watch, I told myself, not a warning. But then the sirens started. Looking carefully into my rearview mirror, I waited for the right moment to do a U-turn, then sped home where a new wave of sirens was going off. Continuously.

Over the next hour, the sirens were constant, wave after wave like a collective MRI blaring through us all. Ken, just home from work, got on the computer to study radar and multiple weather sites while also talking on the phone with Daniel. Rotation just to the west of here. It would be here in less than 30 minutes.

I was on my phone with just about everyone local I knew having the same conversation: "You in your basement?"

"Not yet, you?"

"Not yet either but I'm ready. Got the cat down there already and some blankets."

"Oh, I need to get my kitty downstairs. Talk with you later."

I ran Shay, who was unusually quiet although thunder was his Kryptonite, to the basement and put him behind the door of what we call the way-back, the small storage room between the walk-out part of the basement and the crawl space. With a cat in each elbow and the phone crooked in my neck while I kept talking with everyone, I ran to the way-back part of our basement to deposit more animals.

I closed the door to the way-back, all the animals safely behind it, and rushed upstairs and outside to the deck. "Really?" I said to the dark gray, green and blue-tinged clouds, moving up and over at high speed. Was this going to be the big one? Was this really happening just three weeks before the cancer surgeries? Destruction felt redundant, but I was stubbornly self-centered in seeing this as a personal insult.

Daniel called back, his father's son, furiously tracking the weather, but his mom's son too, near hysteria. "It's massive, Mom, and it's coming right for the house. You have to get in the basement now! You have to get Dad down there too."

I looked for Ken, who was on the western edge of our front deck with a pair of binoculars. Whatever was coming was rain-wrapped (such tornados are hard to see), unusual for this area, so looking west, we just saw a black sky with tinges of dark green.

"Get Dad downstairs now!!!" Daniel screamed into my ear.

"Ken, we need to get downstairs!"

"We have time," he said calmly, adjusting the binoculars. It was still hard to discern any cone-like shape surging eastward toward our hill.

"It's almost there! I can see it on radar!" Daniel yelled. "GET DOWNSTAIRS NOW!"

"Ken! Ken!" He didn't answer me.

I hung up on Daniel and went to grab Ken, who pulled away and yelled, "I know what I'm doing, Caryn. Back off!"

All his life, he had waited to see a tornado and so far had mostly spied wisps of funnels. A lover of weather and adept at predicting it, wherever he went, the tornado went the other way. Years ago, when our kids were little—Natalie an infant and Daniel a toddler, both asleep in their backseat carseats—we were driving south to catch a tornado just ten miles away. Then, paused at a stop sign, we looked into the backseat, sighed, and turned around.

The last time we experienced this was shortly after I completed chemo in 2002. When Ken asked what I wanted to save, I shrugged and suggested the animals, kids, and photo albums, but let the rest go. That tornado lifted back up, veered north, and didn't touch us.

"Ken! Ken! Ken!" By now, I was crying, shaking, and screaming. "Come downstairs! It's almost here!" Daniel was calling me again although I wasn't answering. "Please," I added.

"I know what I'm doing," he answered without looking at me. Maybe this cancer was just too much for him this time after all we'd been through with the last one.

"Please. I don't want to lose you!" I was gulping so hard I couldn't breathe easily, my throat dry and my stomach surely trying to leave my body. But he wouldn't budge He couldn't.

The sirens reached a fever pitch, and I ran back into the house, grabbing my bottle of water, and raced down the stairs to the basement to the way-back where the animals waited. Holding onto Shay as I soaked my dog with my tears, I trembled against the back cement

wall, the winds starting to shake the house, and there, outside in the
big yonder, the love of my life, refusing to come inside. I hated him. I
loved him. I couldn't stand this. I couldn't stand him.

But then he was here, racing in beside me, and before I could say
anything, he pointed to a tight space under some wooden shelves. "Get
in there!" he said.

"No way am I getting in there!" My claustrophobia still full force, I
wasn't going to ride this out stuffed into a dark corner with no light or
space.

We held onto each other and the dog. The sound passing over was
not like the train they tell you a massive tornado sounds like, but more
like loud wind, multiplied by 100. The house creaked. The walls held.
The dog sunk low to the cold concrete. The cats slept effortlessly on
boxes of camping equipment as if it were just another occasion for a
family nap.

It was a minute or two or ten. It was the longest breath I ever took.

Then it was over. Ken pulled me to my feet, and we walked outside.
The house was still there, the trees relatively okay—although some
had branches hanging vertically. There were bundles of leaves on the
ground. And both our phones were ringing.

The tornado just missed us, downing and twisting trees a quarter of
a mile north. But it grew larger and stronger as it blew northeast, overtaking the Pendleton Farm. While they were safe in their basement, the
home and farm were leveled or leaning hard toward the ground. Later,
people would come out of the woodwork for them and for our other
neighbors who lost roofs, windows, whole houses, and certainly a sense
of safety in the world.

Ken and I held each other and cried before answering our phones.
We argued and yelled, cried some more, and both of us were convinced
we had done what we needed to before the tornado. We didn't agree,
and years later, we still don't agree that Ken should have come downstairs earlier, or I should have backed the fuck off. But this is nothing
compared to the suffering of others from this tornado.

Over sixty homes, many within half a mile of ours, were flattened or
lost roofs, garages, or even were themselves damaged—eighteen people were injured in a mile-wide F4 tornado. The F4 part means it had

winds between 207-260 mph, and it's generally the most destructive tornados we see (F5 tornados, with winds up to 318 mph, are pretty rare).
Just a tenth of a mile north of us, on the family land and near Ken's
parents' home, some large trees were hanging broken over themselves.
There was a litter of large and small branches blocking our driveway,
so we climbed out of the car and lifted them away, then went to town.

We drove back home sobered by the power of nature, which was
likely turbo-charged by global warming into larger tornados. The
downed trees and power lines, the flattened small or large houses, the
sirens still going off in many corners of town and country—all reminded us of what our home had survived.

As we walked into our bedroom, out of the corner of my right eye,
blurred as hard rain but also with tears at the moment, I saw the peonies quietly shining into the world. I bent down and inhaled them.

6
Prepare to be Unprepared:
Scenes from A Week

I. Miso Soup

"Prepare to be unprepared," Nomi told me while we waited to order at my favorite Japanese restaurant. This pithy phrase spoke to just about everything I know about cancer treatment, which often feels like a too-fast or too-slow medical excursion in brambly woods with a small bottle of water and no map. Then again, this also speaks to life in general.

Nomi was my former therapist in what felt like another life back in the early 1980s, when I had just moved to Lawrence, and she was offering Bowen Family Systems therapy. The therapy focused on generational patterns and issues, helping us see ourselves in the mosaic of our families of origin and the generational turtles all the way down.

While charting out family history—anniversaries of deaths and divorces, fights and reconciliations—I came to respect Nomi's wisdom. It was no wonder that years later she started a Buddhist meditation group following the teachings of Thich Nhat Hanh. Between me occasionally attending the meditation sessions and her sometimes coming to services at my synagogue, we became fast friends over thirty years, beyond the therapist-patient bubble.

Now she was recounting her own eye healing journey, caused by an epiretinal membrane (also called a macular pucker) that led to years of cataract surgeries, laser procedures, and bumps in the road. "How did you cope?" I asked her right after we ordered.

"It was expensive, but every time my eyesight changed, I got the best new glasses I could. I think I changed prescriptions seven times in two years."

"Did you think it would ever settle down?"

"I didn't know. You know how that is."

The road trips of our senses are full of flat tires as well as roadside stands selling the best sweet corn in the world. There are also long backups for construction that none of us could see coming.

I was nervous about whether I could navigate my upcoming surgical road trip with my triple-sized anxiety, revved up from my backseat-driver, my earlier cancer. Obviously, I had residual issues even if I thought I had thoroughly written, cried, walked, dreamt, and healed my way through the last round with the Big C.

What was I afraid of? Death. That's all, but actually, that's not all. I was deathly scared of pain and being pent up in cages of suffering, depression, and, if it came to pass, a hospital room for five days. My mind kept spinning scenarios of sneaking to the gray hospital stairwell and making a break for it even for just a few minutes of touching the earth. I would need to feel the breeze, smell the impending thunderstorm, even swat at the incessant mosquitos if I were to heal.

"You know, I just bought some stuffed animals from The Toy Store in case I can't leave the hospital," I told her as we each ordered miso soup and sushi. That launched me into telling her the story of that store and its owner, Mike Cnossen. He started the hole-in-the-wall shop on a stretch of Massachusetts Street filled with empty storefronts at the time. It was piles of toys crammed together, but I was still able to wheel in a stroller full of a toddler while carrying Natalie in a front pack to buy some small trinket for Daniel. He was especially dazzled by the stuffed pandas and small cars with tiny doors that opened.

Mike told me this store was his dream, and now here he was, surrounded by Thomas and Friends train sets and Gund stuffed kitties. "I get to make people happy. Kids, but their families too. You step into a toy store, and how can you not smile?"

Less than a decade after opening his dream store, Mike died in a bicycling accident because of a high school driver blinded by the sun. "It's all so arbitrary when we die," I told Nomi, who nodded as the waitress put down our miso soups. But we both knew arbitrary too well.

We looked at each other, her beautiful hazel eyes that had been through so much, taking in the world over so many decades yet able to focus right now on this moment. "This soup is just what I needed," I told her.

"Me too," she said as we smiled.

2. Odin's Eye

An old man turtle needed a name, so I thought hard. I was sitting by a small fountain on a side table in Dr. Sandal's office waiting room, staring at Ben's text and focusing in on the green and yellow tiled pattern of the turtle's shell. What to call him? Then I texted Ben a name: Odin.

It was the same name that came to me for the father of my main character in my novel *Miriam's Well*, my Forrest-Gump-Meets-The-Red-Tent story of the Old Testament Miriam wandering America from the late 1960s onward. Odin was unduly kind, tall, generous, and calm, and he felt like an old friend of mine as soon as I started writing him. He revealed himself to be one of those rare people who don't need any outside validation and truly act as if they're alive to hold lanterns in the dark for the rest of us.

Dr. Sandal came toward me, extending his hand to pull me up, and we went to the consulting room, where we sat facing each other in plush tan chairs. There, I regaled him with updates from the doctors, although I kept forgetting the names of procedures. He nodded patiently.

"But what's on your mind now?"

"Actually, Odin the turtle." I showed him about Ben's text.

"Do you know who Odin is?"

"Yeah, the beloved father of the main character in my novel, *Miriam's Well*."

Dr. Sandal leaned back, tilted his head a bit to the right, and filled me in on more. Odin was the Norse father of the gods. He lost an eye in an interaction with a trickster. "He was a figure at the juxtaposition of wisdom and mythology," he added.

He had a magic eye, I thought. Maybe this is how it grows itself into being although I didn't know how this would play out at the intersection of my story and vision.

Dr. Sandal waited a beat, then leaned forward, raising his eyebrows, the continued, "What you fear is not what you think it is."

I took a long breath, then was overtaken by panic. "But I was working so hard on being healthy," I complained to Dr. Sandal, who, for four years, helped me find my way beyond chronic illness, cycles of antibiotics, and over-the-counter symptom soothers. I slumped down in the plush beige chair of his office, distraught over what I must have done wrong since, like in many of us, self-blame dies hard.

"This cancer was likely in your body for a long time. Some cancers first begin fifteen to twenty years before we know of them." I was amazed, awed, confused, and a little relieved.

A clearing between tangles of self-blame encompassed me. "I guess I just need to breathe, especially when I'm scared, not that we're not breathing all the time."

"Breathing is prayer," he said.

3. Lima Bean

Kris and I met at Wheatfields for almond croissants before heading to Kansas City where Dr. Desai would measure the tumor. Then she and Dr. Patel could order the right configuration of radiation embedded in the gold disk. Before we got to Kris's car, I noticed a small shop on 9th Street full of gourmet rocks. "Do we have a minute?" I ask her.

I opened the wind chime-alerting door and went straight to small green stone turtle. "That's perfect. That will protect you," Kris said. So I got the turtle and placed it in a small interior pocket of my purse, where she slept quietly for a year.

An hour later Dr. Desai raised her eyebrows at meeting Kris, yet another friend or family member. Then it was time to go with Phil to the land of Mordor and lounge on the table so he could massage my eye with the cushy ultrasound joystick.

"You have a lima bean in your eye," Kris told me as she watched the screen. A lifetime as a visual artist—ceramics, fiber arts, paper making, and more—she had an eye for seeing the possibilities in things, even tumors. I wished it were a smaller bean, a navy bean or a lentil, but this was what I was dealt.

As soon as Dr. Desai explained that there was no change in size of the lima bean, she looked away from her computer screen and took my hand. "I promise you, it's going to be okay."

She said a lot more about when to arrive, no vitamins for five days before surgery, and other instructions, but I kept grabbing hold of the life buoy of eight words: "I promise you, it's going to be okay."

Afterwards, Kris and I took my lima bean and the rest of me to Bo Lings, where I watched the psychedelic (because my eyes were dilated) lights of a glass-walled bar change from red to turquoise to purple. Because it was happy hour and we were happy, we ordered all appetizers, including fried eggplant, miniature shrimp rolls, and sturdy crab rangoons of nirvana.

"I promise you," Kris said holding up an egg roll like a pointer, "It's going to be okay."

4. Dreaming the Dragon

Two nights before surgery, sleeping with my real cat and stuffed cat between Ken and me, my stuffed dog on my pillow while the real dog slept on his bed at the foot of ours, I dreamt of a dragon. The brown-scaled dragon wasn't mean or aggressive, just confused a little about being in my dream.

No need to slay the dragon, I realized. It was just passing through, maybe even irrelevant or only temporary. I looked into his brown eyes, and he turned into Shay, who was standing right there, smiling and panting because he wanted to go out, and as always, he was hungry.

In the days leading up to my high noon surgery on June 14th, I realized how little I knew about what I was preparing for. I understood that the implant would be removed June 19th, then the tumor would partially dissolve over the coming months, but there was so much I didn't know. I hadn't met anyone who had had this procedure or rare cancer (1 in 100,000), which gave me a dazed and daunting sense of reality. Would it feel merely uncomfortable or painful? Would I still be me while harboring a radioactive time machine?

I knew such questions are based on a false premise: that there are relevant answers to be had for anything, which is the cost of obsession. When I was first diagnosed with breast cancer, I assured myself that I would simply do what my mother and aunt did: a lumpectomy with a side of radiation. Other people's breast cancer stories reinforced this expectation. All of this worked like scaffolding, lifting me up to high windows to peer into a supposed future, giving my trembling feet a false sense of solid ground. But what happened, like what happens for most of us (even when the treatment turns out to be what we expected), was totally different.

There's nothing like embodied experience compared to reality. My breast cancer was more advanced than I thought. Chemo, which I previously believed was something I would never ever do, turned out to be relatively okay, with occasional steroid-fueled forays into surprise ailments: projectile vomiting, staying up all night re-organizing every closet in the house, and falling asleep in the middle of conversations. Surgeries were moment-by-moment adventures of surrender and recovery, fear and triumph, thirst and replenishment, sometimes with throwing up on a nurse afterwards, a bit of pain, or a rash (turns out I'm allergic to morphine). I was repeatedly dazzled by the body's ability to heal, but even more so by the many ways our friends and community supported our family in the fourteen months between the initial diagnosis and final surgery.

My previous experience didn't mean much when it came to any predictability except for this: the way ahead is made of mystery, love, magic, and more healing than I could have fathomed. I happily took in all the prayers coming my way, whether from Christians invoking Jesus in New Jersey, Jews singing the Mi Sheberach in Kansas, or Buddhist Zapatistas chanting in South America.

This time there was also the steady presence of all my beloveds holding me. Every day on my phone Harriet sent cartoons of dogs sending kisses or texts checking in on me. My mother called regularly to ask how I was. Forest dropped by after work with unsold giant blueberry muffins employees were free to take home. Judy listened to me freak out over wasabi soba noodles at a downtown restaurant right before Kelley met me at another place for the best coconut cream pie in Kansas. Gifts, poems, and love notes showed up in my mailbox and on my front porch.

I spent most of my days in continual birdsong. Each night, I stood on the back deck with Ken behind me, his hands on my shoulders as we thanked the ancestors and land for all the guidance we found there. I sometimes spoke aloud my wishes to get through this, live a long and good life, and with Ken, find the vision and courage to save this land. As Ursula had taught me, I asked for the surgery to be successful, all the doctors and technicians and nurses at their best, and my recovery complete. I prayed for the deepest healing not just from this surgery or this cancer but for my whole life.

But sometimes my paw got caught in the clutch of big-teethed fear, especially when I thought about how this was a medium-to-large tumor. "Don't get married to what you're told," Valerie had said, words I carried in my locket of hope.

There was a dragon, but he wasn't here to hurt me. He was just lost, like me, but we would find our way home.

7
"God's Got You, Baby"

That's what Cynthia said as she led me back to the surgery prep room when I told her I was scared. "And don't you worry because God made women stronger so we can get through anything." Cynthia worked for St. Luke's hospital in Kansas City, and although I didn't know her official capacity, she wore a bright blue button that said, "Success Coach." Her words were cool water to me in a drought, pretty literally because I was parched from the no-water-before-surgery rule.

"I'm so glad to see you," I said as if we were old friends already. She tilted her head toward mine, said, "Uh huh," then looped her black arm in my white one as she escorted me back to the prep room. She was about my height but rounder and completely sure God had both of us in hand. Over the next few hours, she checked on me regularly, teasing me about going to the restroom so often instead of scolding me because I was hooked up to IVs and monitors. But her words about how God's got me helped me breathe just a bit more deeply.

All of us don't resonate with the word "God" or any higher power, but I believe that someone has got us. Call it the higher self. Call it the life force. Call it the Great Spirit. Call it Jesus or Buddha or pure love or real life. For me, God works just fine, shorthand for "the force that through the flower drives the green fuse" (to quote Dylan Thomas) as well as for the unconditional, abiding love we're capable of giving and receiving.

Besides being got by God, I had company, a dream team welcomed to the prep room to sit in a row: Kelley, Judy, Ravi, and Ken, four nervous peas in a pod. Although I had had more than my share of surgeries before—big-time events to cut off my breasts or remove my

uterus, ovaries, and some apron-like appendage—this surgery scared
the bejesus out of me. Maybe it was because I knew so little about this
cancer and its treatment. Maybe it was a gut feeling of what was ahead,
or simply because eyes are delicate creatures best hidden under lids or
behind glasses. We don't envision (so to speak) any part of our eyeballs
cut into to any good end.

"You will arrive at and travel your path," Valerie had told me in
our last session. At the time, it seemed true. But now the what-ifs had
formed a union and were marching through my frontal lobe. On one
hand, I could tell them that even death, as far as I had glimpsed and
believed, was not an end, but what did I know, lying on this table right
now? I thought of another image Valerie gave me about how cater-
pillars have to fight their way out, and that fight makes them strong
enough to use their wings. Would my wings be strong enough?

Kelley reminded me of what she said earlier: see the five days between surgeries as a healing hibernation, a way to tell others "get the
hell away!" while laughing hysterically and reaching for another book I
loved or another pad to color on with my new colored pencils. It could
be a time of deep rest. Judy smiled at me, took my hand, said she knew
I would be all right. Ravi said he was going to go home right now to
make a brisket that I might want to eat later. Ken, weary but trying to
smile, just looked into my eyes.

Dr. Desai strolled in smiling, "You've got everyone here today," she
said. She gave the nurse permission to start the calm-the-fuck-down
drugs. The old friend Versed and its sidekick fentanyl might just erase
some memory tracks, which was fine with me.

I remember Ken kissing me on the lips and everyone filing out
with "I love yous" flying like paper planes through the room. I remember Cynthia holding my hand. Then being wheeled down the hallway,
headfirst, an upside-down sensation, to the very, bright and crowded
room with Dr. Desai, the radiologist, and the anesthesiologist, whom I
had some business with. I asked him to read the note safety-pinned to
my gown, "You will heal easily, quickly, and completely."

"I'm happy to do that," he said, "But I have something else I do. I
ask people to go to a place that they love."

"Yes, yes, let's do that too," I told him. I remembered a cabin we once stayed at near Salida, Colorado, where I sat on a worn lounge chair. Just beyond my bare feet, the perfectly round pond reflected the aspens and cottonwoods, the blue sky, and the one mountain bluebird crossing to perch near me. I made a note to return there later this summer, after it was all over. To actually travel to the future beyond this moment, this state, this lower altitude. The top of my head lit and expanded as if my forehead was breathing in starlight.

Then I was gone.

When I came to, I was going home. "It was so close," Dr. Desai said, and weeks later, she would tell me I was just on the line of being too radioactive, but it turned out that Cynthia was right. God got me, and God got me home.

On the way home I must have sat in the back seat to be as far away from Ken as possible, and we may have talked, but I don't remember anything about the distance between surgery and walking into the house on that rainy afternoon. I found a beautiful vase full of flowers from my sister-in-law Karen and her daughters. There was fresh chicken noodle soup in the refrigerator and homemade bread on the table from my sister-in-law Sandy. There was a box on the table full of fruit and chocolate from Laura. The cats and dog, none of whom I was allowed near, all wanted to wrap around me while Ken herded them another direction.

There was also my bed and how good it felt to sink into it right after looking into the mirror to see my face, half covered with the lead bandage, a diagonal silver blotch. It didn't seem like you should be able to wrap lead around a face, but with dozens of strips of duct tape, everything is possible. Clear tape crisscrossed my face too, reinforcing the duct tape. In fact, all that wasn't covered was my left eye, most of my nose, my mouth, and a segment of my left cheek. I looked like a bad homemade Halloween custom of David Bowie's Ziggy Stardust without the glitter.

We had directions about how to apply new bandages and why. Given the radiation emitting from me, it would be best if I could do this myself. We were also outfitted with gauze, tape, ointments, and printouts of detailed instructions, but all I could do was dump all that on the side of the bed where I would be sleeping in a few minutes.

What followed was a time out of time, mostly spent on the front porch, with the cat scratching at the inside window leading to the porch. The dog tried to open the rickety screen door from the outside, then, failing to get any traction, slumped to the floor while staring mournfully at me.

I opened Pema Chodron's *When Things Fall Apart* to a random page and read, "Nothing ever goes away until it has taught us what we need to know." She went on to explain how new manifestations of our lessons teach us how to open up instead of closing down, how to come out of our shells instead of retreating into them. I thought of turtles and how they could only go forward by extending their necks out into the daring world. Then I opened my computer.

Although I couldn't wear my glasses easily over the bulk of lead and bandages, I could prop them on the tip of my nose and squint just enough to see the screen. My left eye, devoid of its mate, cried sometimes in confusion, but ever the trooper, rallied to help me read Facebook comments under my diagonally divided face.

In the evenings, I could watch, mostly lying on the couch with a bag of frozen peas over my eye because my head hurt, episodes of *Northern Exposure* and imagine myself living in the fictional Cicely, Alaska.

My right eye itched, burned, and ached. My face looked like a young child abandoned at the mall, then beaten up and thrown in a corner. I sat on the porch, sweating in the daytime, sometimes shivering at night, with Ken just on the other side of the door in his chair.

"What's new?" I asked.

"You can't believe the amount of hackberry butterflies out there right now. Also, the daisy fleabane and yarrow in the backyard are starting to bloom." He paused. "So what's new with you," he asked, cracking a smile.

I turned toward him and said I was counting the minutes until I could take more migraine medicine.

"Just sit here and let the wind and birds take care of you," Ken said as he pulled a chair a few inches closer to the screen door.

"You're right," I said, closing my laptop and exhausted left eye, and leaning back. The air buzzed with carpenter bees. "Hey, did you talk to the kids yet?" He nodded, having updated all three although Forest, coming out most evenings to walk the dog and check on me from a distance, was already in the loop.

My temples started pounding, so we stopped talking and I returned to staring into space. I remember reading poet Rainer Maria Rilke about how we teach ourselves and our children to name what's in the space around us—tree, bird, car, streetlamp—rather than see the whole of space itself. In the eighth *Duino Elegies* (translated by Stephen Mitchell), he writes how all other animals see into the open spaces: "Only *our* eyes are turned/ backward, and surround plant, animal, child/ like traps, as they emerge into their freedom." There's something about all this naming that aims our eyes toward the distinctions, at the same time dimming our ability to see beyond what we name.

This small, transitory life passed as I sat quietly as the cacophony of birdsong lit up, muted, or was amplified by the constant wind. The sun's heat was turned to high in mid-June, but sweating made me feel like a creature of summer instead of being just a human with radiation in her eyeball. The cardinals yelled to each other from the Osage orange and walnut trees. A dragonfly floated right outside the screened porch, blending with Ken's black car when it turned upward. I was also floating in this sea of air, lost in another dimension.

Hours later, in the dark bedroom, when another migraine woke me up at 3 a.m., I gave up on taking any more of the hydrocortisone I had been prescribed, which didn't touch the pain but made me nauseous. Instead, I slipped to the basement where we had wisely lined most of the walls with bookshelves when we built the house. Although it hurt to read the titles, I decided to alphabetize all the novels and poetry collections. The only problem was that my head hurt so much I had to repeatedly sing myself the ABC song to remember what came after O or if it was UV or VU. Yet putting the books in order gave me a splash of satisfaction, especially grouping together books by authors I loved from Louise Erdrich to William Stafford.

Then it was back to bed at daybreak. I stopped at the freezer—recently cleaned out and organized to perfection by Anne, who had dropped by last week to help me prepare for surgery—to choose one of my growing collections of ice packs and frozen vegetables. I usually went with peas or a mushy ice pack, and I chose one of each, relishing the idea of going to sleep immediately. But then digestive hell, one of the four (or more) horsemen of surgery aftermath, galloped in with a vengeance, and it was off to the bathroom where I willed myself awake in between clutching my lower belly. Likely it was the anesthesia moving on down the pike.

By the time I was done, I was too awake although my left eye begged to be closed. So I went to the porch, lay on the futon couch, and let dawning birdsong sweep through in the mercy of recovery. I thought of Cynthia's words while I balanced the frozen peas on my forehead. I felt more like a tree or rock than a human, something inert lying relatively still, dappled by the rain, swayed by wind.

In the coming days, there were other moments that buoyed me. When my mother's voice conveyed to me that I was still me. When Judy and Ken carefully rescued a green caterpillar caught against the screen porch screen so it could go on to transform into whatever butterfly it was to become. When Kris dropped off a big box of Ritz crackers, which were the perfect comfort for nausea. When Joy called, her laughter a carnival of happiness on the other end of the phone. When Kelley showed up with chicken soup, the only thing I could imagine eating at the moment. When I talked with Natalie on the phone while spying two elegant tree frogs clinging to the outside of a living room window. When Ken and I laughed together around our cat re-enacting the killing of a hair tie each night to entertain us and garner applause. When I blessedly fell asleep again on the porch to the tune of unseen birds chatting up other unseen birds.

I could only hope others going through challenges, particularly those in chronic pain that keeps unfolding in unpredictable or same-old-same-old ways, have such support holding you, which makes me think of this Rilke poem, "Autumn," which reminds us that we're all falling all the time, "And yet there is Someone, whose hands/ infinitely calm, holding up all this falling."

God's got me, I told myself, as I prepared for more of the unpreparable: the surgery to remove the radiative gold heart. I didn't know if I'd see Cynthia, but I wrapped her words around me like a woven shawl of the blue and green stories of leaves in a tropical forest, and prayers sung by a woman who had seen it all from half-way up a mountain we had all climbed.

8

The Pain of Light

"I love you," I told the anesthesiologist and nurse when they started me on fentanyl, and I meant it. By the end of the five days of hosting radiation, the pain in my head flashed so violently that I was awake in agony all night. But once I got to the prep room, told the good people around me of my nausea and migraines, all manner of relief ensued. The pink-faced young nurse with blue-green eyes gave me a small cotton ball with peppermint oil to smell for my nausea, then inserted additional meds into my IV. The anesthesiologist, who looked like he ran marathons between surgeries, gave me a Tylenol, then okayed the heavier narcotics, which proved to be miraculously fast-acting. In the queendom of the body, peace and joy rose over all the land like a tangerine sunrise.

I vaguely remembered the drive to the hospital while our friend Rabbi Levin prayed for me on speaker phone, speaking the words of the Misheberech, the healing prayer. The pain was a pair of scissors dividing me from myself, and I couldn't participate in anything that seemed like a conversation, although Ken did a good job of thanking him. I tried to say "thanks," but no words would come. I remember three other moments pain divided me from language, each time in the later stages of labor when I also couldn't endure anyone so much as patting my shoulder.

While Ken parked the car, I raced to the waiting room to look for Cynthia, but everyone I encountered was not-Cynthia. I started to cry as I checked in at the desk with someone efficient but also pretending not to see a bandaged-faced woman weeping. As I collapsed into a chair, a hand landed on my left shoulder. "Cynthia!" I called out, which made me cry harder, not a good move when you have a lead patch over your eye.

"Oh, Baby, how are you?" she asked.

"Not good," I gulped, trying to calm myself while standing up to face her.

She put her other hand on my other shoulder and looked me in my one uncovered eye. "You remember what I told you?" I nodded. "See, I told you God's got you, and look at you, standing up and walking back in to get this over with. You're okay, Baby." I lost it more while she hugged me before heading off to her next patient. Then I cried harder because she knew how radioactive I was, and she still held me tight.

By the time they wheeled me into the surgery room, I was feeling no pain. Just like with childbirth (although I wasn't medicated for that), I was looking forward to getting the thing out of me as quickly as possible. I harbored no understanding yet that this wasn't the end of treatment but the beginning of a long recovery with many chapters time would write on my body. "I was very worried about the collateral damage of all the radiation," Ken would tell me later, and he had good reason.

I remember even less of what happened after this surgery except the relief of just a bandage over my eye under a miniature oval-shaped colander, and praying for the AC to come on faster as soon as I got into the car. I fantasized about picking up the cat, heading back to my bedroom with Shay at my heels, and lying down for a long time.

The next day, once Dr. Desai removed the bandage, I discovered I couldn't tolerate light, especially from my new mortal enemy, the sun. Driving home, I had to pattern together a new normal: two pairs of sunglasses with a towel over my head so that I could only look down at my confused hands. Walking car to house, the white-hot sun was a cruel seeker, bleeding through everything to make my eyes and head ache. But thankfully, there was the possibility of cool and dark places, where I burrowed for the rest of the day.

The next morning, Ken distracted me by reading aloud an article on asteroids from *Science News*. Forest dropped by to give me more leftover lemon muffins from work. Friends called or I called them. Yet when pain persisted, even a fresh sleeve of Ritz crackers and a stiff iced tea did little to distract me.

I could never imagine slapping a kitten or stealing a car, but my mind, along with the rest of me, would conjure up freezing mountains for pain relief, and god knows what sins I would be capable of along the way. When I consider the times in my life when pain ruled the roost—those three natural childbirths, an upper G.I. bleed once, and a history of migraines since I was a teenager—I know I would easily beg at the altar (or gutter) of pharmaceuticals for anything to take that pain away, and if that wasn't possible, put me to sleep until it was over.

I've been a lucky body for the most part on the pain spectrum. I thought of people who live with chronic pain—constant back agony, heart-numbing depression, myriad shooting pains throughout the body without rhyme or reason. There's also the pain of the social body born of prejudices and biases: constant attacks for not being white or straight or thin or whatever else. At the time of my surgeries, migrant children were being locked in cages without food or bedding, alone or crowded without enough ventilation or tenderness to survive without incurring damage. We may not be experiencing such pain directly, but that's the thing about pain. Knowing it intimately can tilt open the door of our own heart so that we can choose to respond to the pain of others.

For about six weeks, I was pain's constant companion. But perspective tells me it's just a drop in the fuck-it bucket of what so many others are going through right now, whether it's a six-year-old Guatemalan boy trying to keep a toddler brother fed on a concrete floor in Texas, a neighbor down the street carrying the shattered pieces of her grieving heart to an empty bed, or someone who cuts me off in traffic because he was up most of the night with stabbing shoulder pain.

"Oh, for the relief from pain!" is an animal chorus, coming back around at every turn. "May we be free of suffering and the root of suffering," goes one of the primary Buddhist prayers. So much pain begets ripples of greater pain, often without resolving the original pain or with replacing it with something even more vexing.

But not all pain can be relieved. Some of the Turning Point writers live with sharp or dull pain from years of harsh chemotherapy or progressive neurological disease. Some of my friends, surviving without beloved partners or parents or children, carry the fullness of acute and searing emptiness with them daily. Some of the people who brush past me in the food co-op or bank are hurting in an alphabet of agony most people can't imagine.

All we can do is say, *We're hurting.* All we can ask, sometimes just with our silence: *Please help,* or *please just sit here with me cursing this moment of sharp edges.* All we can tell ourselves is maybe tomorrow will be better even if we're still repeating this refrain tomorrow. All we can give are the words *I love you* to the world.

Meanwhile there was the light, usually a happy thing, a sign of hope or even joy, hurting me. There was my smart-ass head, my acute-to-the-splendid-details-of-the-living-earth eyes, my look-on-the-bright-side outlook all wounded in this underground bunker. During a potluck at our house with friends of Daniel's, I sealed myself off in our bedroom, yet another bag of frozen peas on my forehead and the ceiling fan in high gear on this sweltering day. One of Daniel's pals knocked on my door, tilted it open, and softly said he was leaving a small bag of edibles in the freezer for me in case I needed them. I cried at his gesture.

There was also Laurie, a dear friend and healer who combines acupuncture, energy healing, and craniosacral therapy to treat people after retiring from years of work as a chiropractor. We connected at one of my workshops a year ago and became fast friends, especially since she lived near Dr. Desai's office. At the beginning, in the middle, and after those six weeks of intense pain, Ken and I aimed our old CRV up her steep drive on the Kansas side of State Line Road (Missouri on the other side of the street).

While Ken visited with Luna, her guardian spirit husky, downstairs, I lay on the massage table upstairs with an eye pillow covering my eyes. We joked about realizing that we didn't need to be so hard on ourselves as she stuck needles in my ankles, wrists, and top of my head. Sometimes a sting, but it faded in a breath—acupuncture has been a friendly therapy for me for years, and true to form and to Laurie's gifts, the pain in my temples receded.

So much deep relief poured through my shivering body that my right eye started crying and wouldn't stop. Luna howled from downstairs in tune with my liberation.

9

Shut Up and Close Your Eyes

Like Dracula, I had to forgo direct sunlight. As July turned up the heat and multiplied the humidity, I burrowed deeper into the dark, so far from my natural habitat. But there's nothing like pain and healing to guide an anxious mind out of its usual hamster cycles and into the present.

For a person who loves reading, movies, watching videos of *Oklahoma* on Broadway, and staring into the layered foliage to find the bird responsible for all the racket, I was disoriented. But for all ills, there are remedies, and the best one I discovered started about 8:30 p.m. on the night porch as dusk traveled dark. It took a while for me to stop resisting what this body was telling me in no uncertain terms: shut up and close your eyes.

In a Kansas summer, twilight comes calling with thousands of extras. Sitting out there with Ken, we counted at least six different kinds of cicadas, starting with the low soft click of the green-winged cicada, then the back-and-forth mild buzzsaw of Tibicen bifidus. Eventually, we got to the steady sweet roar of the plains cicada, which sounded like wheels of a wagon moving across the prairie although the wheels, spokes, and wagon were made of cicadas, and of course, hauling cicadas.

Tree frogs leapt into the fray for short or long stretches. Crickets showed up as they always do when it comes to getting any party started. Thousands of insects and amphibians not only coordinated their wild rushes into circle hums or steady chirps of green joy with their fellow specie comrades, but blended their sounds into something both beyond and encompassing the essence of music. Plains cicada stretched their

journey song into multiple cycles, then stopped. Chuck-will's-widow, a
brown-speckled bird with a flat head and lizard-like coloring, jumped
in the gap with curvy whistles, then paused. Suddenly, everyone from
every direction, it started again.

We listened, my dreams merging with what I heard as I dozed in
the chair. I wanted to lie down to sleep in the house, but Ken urged
me to wait for the telltale call of night, heralded by the katydid. "When
will the katydids start?" I asked, and just then, katydid whispers circled
over us. "Listen carefully," he said. "There are two katydids," which
we quickly named Katy Did and Katy Didn't because that's what they
sound like.

"I keep thinking about the farm," Ken told me.

"I dreamt about it last night. There were invader raccoons trying to
eat our house, but then it wouldn't stop raining."

"Do you think we should . . . ." He stopped. We had done all the
"should" we could imagine to no avail. I knew he was going to ask if
we should contact his aunts, see again if they would agree to dissolve
the trust so that we could buy at least a portion of the land and protect
it.

"Do you want to call your Aunt Wilma just to see what . . . ." I
stopped too. Just asking the question made us both slump more in our
chairs. "You know, if we lost the farm, it's not like it would kill us," I
added.

He sounded unconvinced. Ken was so wedded to this land, but his
love for the earth was stronger. Surely we could plug that love into
another place? I was shocked at the calmness of my thoughts.

"I can't go there," he finally said.

"Like you can't go there with what if this cancer comes back?"

"Uh huh," he said quietly, and then told me to listen to the sudden
loudening of the katydids.

A few nights later, Anne arrived to massage my feet to help me relax and to lessen the pain still holding forth in my forehead. I hugged
her, then we went inside, so that I could lie on the couch, my feet in
her lap as she pressed points correlating with different organs, none
of which were happy to be kerplunked out of the loud rave they were
attending. The sky darkened into a classic summer storm as the three

of us sat facing the southern windows displaying IMAX-quality flashes and slashes of light.

Within a few minutes, the storm hit, multiple strikes of lightning across the stage of the southern sky, thunder that made the dog dive into a corner, and in quick order, darkness. "I love this," Anne said.

"Me too," said Ken.

"Me three," I added.

Then a huge lightning bolt hit to the southwest. Shay, although he was 90 pounds, threw himself across my torso, and all our lights went out without even flickering first. None of us rushed to look for flashlights or candles, and instead, we started laughing until our laughter quieted to awe. It was warm enough, and with the windows cracked open to just a whistling line, tolerable enough without air-conditioning.

We sat in the dark as we all looked south out the five windows framing the dance of lightning strikes. The green shock of a vertical bolt or the white horizontal sizzle strike captivated us, but I started to babble about people we knew before boring even myself. *Listen*, the world said. So I stopped talking.

Yet the peace of the insect and storm symphonics couldn't dampen down the thrashing roar of my mind. It woke me at 4:30 a.m. most days, when I was caught in fretful dreams that sweated into my waking life. I sat up to wake myself out of worry about whatever: how to fit my laptop into an antique desk or where to find a pay phone when they hardly exist anymore. But once awake, my mind tripped into worries about climate change as well as how would I wake up early enough for a morning gig next February if I didn't sleep well the night beforehand. My mortality was trolling the outskirts of my consciousness, overseeing dozens of things that could potentially go wrong.

I tried to steer my thinking away from a particular tar pit of habitual anxiety, a well-developed one-act play called "The Farm," that included invading bulldozers like those All-Terrain Armored Transport walkers from *Star Wars*. I got up, stumbled to the hall, turned on the light so that I could find Benadryl to knock me out, and for good measure, some GABA too.

While I wanted to wake Ken up, he didn't need me to add to his jolts of wakefulness. He was worrying about the farm at different hours than me, retreating to the living room to read a book until he got tired enough to return to sleep. Both of our uncertainties over this land and my health were growing that July. Maybe it had something to do with a particularly energetic full moon lately, the reality that we are in the sixth age of extinction with species vanishing daily, and so many people and other species experiencing avoidable suffering born of oppression, greed, arrogance, and ignorance.

The middle of the night breeds little worlds that grow at the speed of darkness into big swaths of panic. Realizing who the little man is behind the curtain didn't help much except to remind me that on the other side of survival, the shit often hits the fan. I have worked enough with people living with serious illness to recognize how, months after being spit out on the beach from the whale of chemo, surgeries or radiation, the terror catches up with us.

Valerie had reminded me that it can be helpful to do a reality assessment when the panic gets off the leash by asking myself if what I feared was really happening at this moment. No? Then what is happening? Judy told me, "So since what I worry about never happens, I don't need to worry about it." But in the middle of that shakiness gripping the center of my belly, I forgot everything until I remembered to aim my thoughts toward slower breaths and less hunger for answers.

I also knew I was far from alone. Friends and family often called out, "Same!" when I told them of a recent running of the bulls in my body and mind. In my visit with Dr. Sandal last week, he told this ancient riddle: "What is the most amazing thing in the world? That everyone is dying and no one believes it." This truth is from ancient India's sacred text, the Mahabharata. Mortality is a kick in the ass, and it makes sense that given how much we live in a death-denying (and at times defying) culture, that sometimes the space between a sense of control and life's fragility fills with adrenalin.

So for all of us who occasionally experience any size panic attacks in any nook and cranny of our lives, it's good to know that we're in honest company. Sometimes there's a quick fix, and often there's not. But there's time, turning us from the temporary into the next temporary. Like all those nights when I got up to sit in the bedroom chair at 4:45 a.m. or 2:11 a.m. or 5:01 a.m. in the dark, telling myself to remember the weather, the sky, the time is always changing.

Then I'd return to bed to watch Ken's back move in and out just a little as he slept on his side in the beautiful healing darkness. I would listen to the hum of the air-conditioner, the snoring of the dog, the padded rush down the halls of the running of the cats. From outside, I could hear the barred owl calling, *who cooks for you?* And like most daytime creatures in the dark, I would eventually close my eyes.

10

Don't Make Eye Contact with the Owls

The two great horned owls blended so well into the craggy foliage near the Colorado pond that I was shocked when I found them staring at me, each the size of a toddler. Their dark eyes pierced my green ones.

"Turn away," Ken said. "Don't keep making eye contact. They'll feel threatened," he said near the cabin I had remembered while going under for surgeries. It was hard to take my one seeing and one not-so-much-seeing eyes off the owls, who were surely so much more cognizant than humans of what was happening in the ultra-focused world of food and danger, prey and predator.

We were here for five days, the same length of my radiation trip, just two months after the ordeal. I had front-loaded several work gigs, including a writing workshop in Greensburg, Kansas, on the way here to make up commitments and income kicked down the road. Greensburg was famous for both a giant hole in the ground, namely what was once the world's biggest hand-dug well, and one of the most destructive tornadoes in history.

In 2007, a 1.7-mile-wide tornado, wider than the city itself, tore diagonally through this town, then stayed on the ground for another 22 miles. Just about everything had to be rebuilt, including the senior center where I did a workshop on writing our life and legacy. The town was a place of big views and tilted young trees, aiming northeast from the southwest wind. New sidewalks still glittered in the sharp sunlight, and new windows shone in the energy-efficient new high school and city hall. Newly-constructed homes lined blocks with such fierce light due to the absence of mature trees that I had to keep my eyes hidden under two pairs of sunglasses and a ball cap.

We drove west the next morning, the altitude increasing in way-out western Kansas, where I always felt freer and lighter. For months and weeks I had been counting down to this trip, the big escape to a place of downright cold temperatures each night, the persistent smell of pine, and breathless treks, even just from the car to a gas station bathroom, because of the altitude. We hadn't been to Colorado in some years, which is just about against the law of physics if you live in Kansas.

Now we were crossing the long wide eastern plains of Colorado, calling out "side luck!" when a train the length of Rhode Island side-traveled the interstate or "over luck!" when we passed under a train on a bridge. Now we were heading into the foothills, arriving in Colorado Springs to see friends Tom and Janet in nearby Manitou Springs. Now we were hugging them goodbye, especially poignant because Tom had late-stage pancreatic cancer. It wouldn't be long now. His sober, loving presence clung to us and his body hugged us more than usual. His eyes looked into ours, saying, *I love you, take care, I'll miss you.*

Now we were crossing South Park, a 10,000-plus-feet-high tundra between mountain ranges, the big bright sky multiplying itself, the mid-day summer temperature only reaching 47 degrees while wind and scraggly trees played across the wide expanse in miniature. Now we were turning south onto Highway 24, side-saddling the Collegiate Peaks until we arrived at the cabin, just west of Salida, one of our favorite Colorado towns.

The cabin was like it was years ago, compact and thick-walled because it was made from straw bales, then stucco-ed over. The interior was painted in pale earth tones with an occasional green or turquoise wall. There was a pile of DVDs from the early 2000s near the TV, and the bedroom held wall-to-wall shelves with board games, children's toys, and old hardcover books.

The pond, which I remembered as sublime, was overgrown with algae and cluttered at its southern edges with floating toys, a broken chaise lounge, a kid's pink plastic scooter. I had romanticized this place, I realized, while circling its overgrowth and clouds of mosquitoes.

But then there was the hot tub, where we held court with the sky each night, leaning back in the water to behold the stars spread in triplicate, the air cooling quick while the hot tub was warming too much. On our first night in the tub, Ken told me about a phone call he had gotten earlier from Aunt Wilma, who had an idea to save the farm. I put my feet in front of some of the jets. We just looked at each other in the dark, immersed in this splendid place in water and starlight, neither of us saying what could or could not happen.

Then it hit me how big this was. "You what? What happened?"

"She was saying the trust could hire a lawyer to dissolve itself, then we could buy the land."

"But how could we afford that?" I asked. For months, I had cut back on workshops, taking on new coaching clients, or teaching classes because my main gig was cancer treatment. The cupboard of our savings was bare after paying so many medical bills, even with good health insurance.

We spun into a circular conversation all too familiar to us about how this was the only way forward, but it seemed impossible. What if we could buy just half the farm and let the other half be sold to developers? But how could we live with losing the whole farm? What if we could only protect the back 40 where our house was? What if, what if, what if?

"Maybe we should imagine that we already saved the farm and now we're figuring out the conservation easement stuff," I offered. We had been checking in with Jerry Jost, the then-director of the Kansas Land Trust, since 2018 when he set up a file for the Wells Farm as a potential conservation easement project. We had contacted him at the same time we made an offer, based on the most recent appraisal of the land, to Ken's aunts shortly after Alice died. Then we tried to be patient as all but one of the trustees approved of it, hoping the last hold-out aunt would change her mind. Sometimes when I ran into Jerry and his wife Deborah walking their handsome black-and-white rescue dog Teddy, I felt a little sheepish about how we had no progress to report on buying the land.

We always knew that if we could buy this place, we would do what we could to put it in a conservation easement.

We had first shared the idea of putting the development rights of the farm in a land trust with Ken's aunts, in the 1990s, shortly after the Kansas Land Trust formed. This nonprofit would protect the land forever. It had been created after the heartbreak over destruction of the Elkins Prairie, a 14,000-year-old prairie on the western edge of Lawrence. The land trust had grown to protect 40,000 acres across over 80 properties (and counting) throughout the state.

The idea of a land trust is that it can negotiate a legal contract—a conservation easement—in which a landowner gives the land trust development rights. In turn, the land trust protects the land in perpetuity, maintaining staff and resources to do periodic check-ups. It ensures that any future owners (since land can still be sold when it has a conservation easement on it) understand what restrictions apply, and takes legal action when owners don't. Along the way, there are restrictions. Owners can't put commercial enterprises on the land, divide it up and sell it, or even build homes outside of a small area defined a building site envelope.

It was a no-go with Ken's aunts, even before they understood this. Aunt Eleanor proclaimed, "We're not giving the government our land." Explaining that we would just be giving away the development rights didn't help. Most of them, born in the lean and mean 1930s, knew poverty as a very visceral experience of their childhoods. Land could keep you safe, give you a place to grow your food, even protect you. Plus, who knows? If tragedy struck, you might need to sell that land to survive or help your family.

Eventually, we got enough letters from Ken's aunt who refused our offer that we had to accept it wasn't going to happen now.

"Do you know how Gordian knots are undone? They can't be untied. They have to be cut through," Ken said as the clouds started rolling in, obscuring the stars. I felt Ken's foot on my left calf.

"Like by a lawyer? Someone who has a background in Gordian knot fuckery?"

"Isn't that what the legal profession is all about at its best?" he said as we climbed out of the tub and toweled ourselves off in the cold air. Neither one of us could sleep well that night, both wondering if we get to keep the farm. When I finally slept, I was lost in a city that was a dream version of New York City but with more traffic and fewer Chinese restaurants.

We got lost other ways. One day, we aimed the CRV up a dirt road that promised a scenic outlook and the start of a trail, but we soon realized the road gave way to rock, long flat slabs, and some were at dramatic angles. "Should we keep going?" we asked each other. It didn't take long before we realized the answer was no, but by then, we couldn't fathom where to turn around. The thing called a road wrapped around the edge of a steep mountain with only enough room for one car. To our right, rock walls towered. To our left, a dizzying drop.

Ken gripped the wheel. He was a good driver, but at this moment, scared also. You choose a road without knowing where it will lead, then this can happen.

As the road got more vertical, we stopped the car, pulled on the emergency brake, and got out to look for options. If we moved a bunch of smaller rocks hugging the crease along a rock wall extending thirty feet up, we might have enough room to make a nineteen-point turn. So that's what we did, hauling rocks the size of bowling balls out of the way, getting back into the car to creep back a foot, then pull forward until we were turned back toward the descent. It took a long time and our hearts beat like hummingbirds'. We crept down at two mph until we reached the turn-off, so relieved that we promptly returned to the cabin to celebrate with PB&J sandwiches.

That night, lying in the hot tub outside the kitchen, staring up into the stars in the cold air, I said I was so glad we didn't die today. Ken put his arm around me. "How in the world can you stand this hot tub?" We laughed, an old joke that I lived for immersing myself in extremely hot water, my body happy to de-evolve back into a water creature.

"How can you not love it?" We looked at each other, our eyes old friends.

"Do you know why I think Orion is a woman?" he asked me.

"What? But Orion wears that big belt."

"I think it's a sash holding a womb, and inside it are billions and billions of stars." Darkness is where things are created, incubated, and we bring our shadows with us, seeing in the dark too.

The next day, taking well-paved roads only, we drove to another destination, one full of big views, strong coffee, and even fresher air, Leadville. A relatively small town at an altitude of over 10,000 feet,

Leadville was a hot spot during the 1860s Colorado Gold Rush. Now it is an extreme mountain sport mecca peopled by artists and loners overlooking the beautiful waters of Twin Lakes and surrounded by 14ers, mountains over 14,000 feet tall.

Being in Leadville was a lot like being on the top of the world. Although I often got headaches, nausea and dizziness at such heights, I sensed this would be different, and it was. We stopped for coffee, and walking into a small rough-wood-walled shop, we immediately saw two old friends from Lawrence, one Forest's speech teacher from when he was six, and Anne's mom. After a lively what-are-the-chances conversation, we shared updates of what we'd seen in the mountains.

Walking out of the coffee shop, I laughed with Ken that even here, old friends converge. Wearing my double sunglasses and cap, plus walking on the shady side of the street because of the fierceness of the sun at this altitude, I headed one direction and he another, promising to meet later at the car. Without planning it, we converged in a bookstore.

Back in the car, after joking about what would have happened if we fell off the mountain yesterday, a remote place where it might have taken a long time to even find the bodies, we got quiet. Our fear was spent past its limit on cancer, and for years before and right now, the farm.

There was nothing more to say. All altitude now, the luminous world a blur or slap for so long, but now there was this stretch of driving from the top of Leadville south to the cabin. In a few days, we would go further east and down in altitude to Denver to see good friends Scotty and Joy, take long walks together, and eat steak and apple pie while talking movies, memoirs, and memories.

Almost dusk, the silver pink-lined clouds to the west, started to dissolve above the Collegiate peaks. The acute pain in the rearview mirror along with the hum of the old car carried us. The bottle of cool water I sipped, then passed to Ken. We were freed from all we had been through this year, so we let the open field of the road lead down the mountain to where the owls would see us, but we wouldn't see them.

11

I Don't Want to Die

What do you do with old fear, the kind that sets up a cot in the basement of your psyche, somewhere between boxes of essays you wrote in college and a giant pressure cooker you'll never use?

This is what I was thinking as I drove home from yoga one late August evening. Ken and I had sweated our way through a lot of standing poses and downward dogs although this wasn't hot yoga, just a humid evening that overcame the air-conditioning. I felt strong for most of the class, especially when I leaned against a wall to do one of my favorite standing positions, half-moon. I love this pose of perpendicular stretching, especially against the friendly backing of a good wall, one foot on the floor, the other lifted at a 90-degree angle, one hand on the floor, and the other reaching for the sky. If it sounds like I'm describing Twister, it's actually the opposite, a way to unfurl and reach all directions at once.

At the end of class, lying in savasana, otherwise known as corpse pose, as Anne spoke in a quiet voice I couldn't make out, fear hopped off its cot and squatted beside me, waiting for me to get up and make it some scrambled eggs.

When I rolled to my right side, then pushed myself up to sit cross-legged, I felt that old scaredy-cat drop in the pit of my stomach. I put my hands together at the center of my chest, said "Namaste" with the other students, then pressed my palms into the wooden floor to say "Namaste" to the earth. But I sure wasn't feeling the divine in me bowing to the divine in anything else.

Ken got his car to go to a meeting while I pulled out of the parking garage a little disoriented about whether to go home, head to the grocery salad bar, or drive across town to get a slice of pizza that would likely make me feel sick later. I aimed for home out of a lack of imagination, drained by the sudden departure of all that half-moon bad-assery expansion.

Driving south on Massachusetts street, I remembered when cancer dread tunneled through me as I sat on the edge of our bed, mid-afternoon on a hot September day in 2002, staring at the overcast sky. Ninety seconds. That's what brain scientists say is the length of a very powerful emotion, but during those ninety seconds, you can easily feel like you're going to dissolve into glue and staples, a mess of contradictions trying to connect into something cohesive.

I stopped at a red light, then turned left to head the long way down Louisiana Street to the country, I was remembering how what I feared was accompanied by lots of loving friends and family who dropped off vegetable soups or sent me funny greeting cards. If I had died from that cancer years ago, it would have been horrendous for me, but I might be gone or reincarnated into a kestrel or I could have found my way to sing alongside old dead friends at some cosmic campfire. What Ken and our kids would experience was so devastating that just the thought made me tremble.

As I turned on my bright headlights to see better in the dark, I thought about the statistics my oncologist Dr. Stein gave me in 2002: 43% survival rate in five years without chemo, 57% with chemo. "Why would he even tell us that?" I asked Ken after leaving the oncologist office back in the spring of 2002.

"He has to. It's probably something all oncologists are required to say." But that was before we learned how little and how much statistics can mean. Do I contradict myself? Like Walt Whitman said, yes, because I contain or am haunted by multitudes, including cancer cells, already in all of us all the time.

To quote one of our favorite movies, *The Shawshank Redemption* in the voice of Morgan Freeman, "Get busy living or get busy dying." Yet there's a distinction between what we might consider regular life ("ordinary people stuff," Dr. Stein used to tell me with delight when I got a bad cold) and extraordinary daily maneuvers through chemo, radiation, surgery, experimental treatments, hospice, palliative care, and other blaring billboards that flash "We're All Gonna Die!"

I've been with many people who have put their statistics to shame—

Teri, who is now over twenty-five years out from being told her Stage Four cervical cancer (with metastases to her lungs and liver) would kill her within months. Janice had late-stage colon cancer that spread to her liver and lungs, and thanks to a clinical trial, she has been fine, thank you, for over twenty years. Linda is still alive although shaky with a bundle of side effects from eighteen years of fending off Stage Four ovarian cancer.

Such statistics can play out the other way too. In my early writing workshops, I worked with two young mothers, one who cheerfully called herself the Edgar Allen Poe of writing depressing poetry and the other who had a rosy outlook on life, growing a lot of her own food with her toddlers in tow. They each died quickly from early-stage breast cancer. Despite the seeming impossibility of it, my aunt and a good friend had their breast cancers return twenty years after diagnosis, although both fared well in fending off the latent cancers.

The numbers aren't meant for human bodies with our delicate tissues and ordinary bones, I realized as I put the car in park and stepped outside, pausing to look up at the cloud cover. I could make out a few stars. I went in the door to put together leftover refried beans, chicken, and rice into a makeshift burrito bowl, remembering what Dr. Stein told me years ago: the stats consider any way you can die, including the unfortunate hit-by-a-bus cliché.

Statistics scoop up the whole population together, including people who aren't able or willing to do regular scans, eat lots of broccoli or blueberries, or avoid chemically-infused foods, stressful occupations, or land. Yet as we all know or should know, being a perfect specimen of a body doesn't ensure survival. In fact, some babies are born with cancer. My friend Nancy reminded me of this once, saying, "How much more innocent can you get?"

On that lovely evening on the porch, as I sat down on with that burrito bowl, I gave in to the voice, surely my father's, telling me that I needed to face reality (as if we know what reality is) and go ahead and research the statistics on this cancer. I knew that people tending to post their own experiences on the interwebs are themselves usually on the desperation bus, sharing worst-case scenarios in search of miracles. But that and all the doctors who adamantly said not to research this didn't stop me.

Something screeched. I wondered if idiots were still igniting fireworks at the overlook even if we were way past the fourth of July. Then it was quiet. I had eaten my dinner mechanically without tasting it. I picked up my laptop from beside me as the crickets started up again. I defied myself and googled "ocular melanoma." The air was gentle and comforting. Shay was licking up the leftovers from my bowl on the floor.

It is a rare cancer, only affecting about six out of a million people, which makes it trickier to get reliable information. I opened each piece of relevant information into a dozen separate tabs, then started reading. The words spelled out low survival odds, lots of suffering and disfigurement, and the word "aggressive" used repeatedly. My temples started throbbing and my breath shallowed.

I closed all the tabs, then the computer. I remembered a conversation with Valerie about my fear of metastases. "I can't sit with this," I told her.

"Anxiety is an asshole," she said, then helped me unpack it with her white board and a marker. "What is happening now?" she asked. I wasn't obviously dying right now. The future was a crap shoot, a karmic spin of the wheel.

I also knew that these tidal waves of fear didn't just come from doom-scrolling but from being in the beginning of the aftermath when a lot of sad birds come home to roost. I had spoken to Natalie recently about how hard it was for her not to be there for my surgeries, even though I wasn't people-worthy at the time. She realized that all she went through as a nine- and ten-year-old watching her mother lose her hair, sleep a lot, and keep coming home with bandages, drains, and small white bags full of prescription meds caught up with her in new ways. "I spiraled," she told me, "tapping into all that childhood stuff with watching you go through cancer."

I hadn't given much thought to how the first cancer, let alone this second one, impacted my kids even if they were supposedly adulted up by now. But what marks us doesn't happen in a vacuum. I wondered how this had colored psyches of all three of our kids, my mother, and close friends just as some of their trials made me grapple more with the slippery slope of life.

I listened to the trees and sky, then got myself up and walked off the porch and into the field. It was dry enough that there were likely few chiggers and fewer ticks, so I kept walking. Clouds were sliding over the almost-full moon, which glowed in that gold pink of its reflected light meeting the ensuing darkness. The land held me.

At this moment, before I would talk with Ken—once again depositing my fear in his tired arms—and before I would down a Benadryl to help me sleep, I said a combination of Lamott's three prayers in one sentence: *I don't want to die.*

12

A Bug in the Ear

Harrison Ford wasn't having it, and in typical Indiana Jones fashion, he climbed up the side of the cardboard box to lunge himself toward escape even if three of us were waiting there to catch him and put him back in the maze. A handsome, large dark green and black turtle, Harrison Ford showed us in quick order that he had no interest in lumbering toward the prize lettuce at the end of the maze Sam, one of Ben's students, had constructed for this experiment.

In fact, only one of the turtles, Alan Arkin, was motivated enough by the call of a strawberry to head toward it in a field north of us where Sam and other students were testing the turtles. Elie Wiesel climbed forward a few steps, then stopped, but you can understand why a turtle with his name and a burn-damaged shell had had enough. Persephone tried to bite her way out and would have succeeded if Sam didn't remove her. Leslie Jones, whom I named after a tiring visit to have my eyes checked after the last surgery, took to knocking over some of the dividers between herself and the strawberries, but you'd expect that from her. Barack Obama, Chewbacca, and Lady of the Lake did well.

Yesterday, I just had my first of ten or more years of quarterly CT scans to ensure the cancer didn't follow my body's maze to lungs or liver. I was shaky going in, two Lorazepams in my system and Christina Perri singing "A Thousand Years" through my earbuds. That song would turn out to be my CT scan soundtrack for the foreseeable future because there's nothing like a musical prompt to tell the body, "You've got this."

That afternoon Ken and I went to see Dr. Soule for one of what we hoped would always be good-news post-scan visits. She had already set up a protocol of scan in the morning and appointment with her early afternoon so that we wouldn't be playing the call-if-it's-good-news, come-in-if-it's-not game. She walked jauntily into the room and said, "Whenever I walk in smiling, it's good news," and it was.

Now it was a day and night later, and after a morning of visiting the turtle races and afternoon while contemplating cleaning the house without actually doing anything, Ken and I were both exhausted. I found myself drifting more quickly than usual into deep sleep. I hadn't slept much the night before the scan out of fear, or the night afterwards because I was too relieved to be able to relax, so I was now finding just the right three bears' bed of rest.

Two hours later, Ken and I learned a new wrinkle of what "in sickness and in health" means as well as a novel use for leftover Manischewitz Passover wine. As with most things, it began with something very small, a bug in my right ear. This one was tiny enough to fit with room for rustling its wings at high speed somewhere near my eardrum.

I woke Ken up. We guessed it was a tiny moth, but it didn't seem to be able to make its way toward the divine mothership of the flashlight he kept shining in my ear.

Unfortunately, we were experienced at luring moths from ears. A few weeks ago, we had implemented Operation Moth-Ear Rescue when a minuscule moth lost its way in the same ear. Natalie, who was visiting at the time, held a flashlight while Ken used tweezers to encourage the little moth out to the light of existence and then out the door after several minutes of moth-wing-rattle in my brain that I hoped never to experience again.

This time, we tried all the old tricks but the critter just burrowed in deeper, making me feel like I was losing my mind as rapidly as it fanned its wings. I freaked out. I had myself a little pity party. I got pissed off and cried. We tried ear shaking at many angles of repose as well as squirting in water to see if the bug would swim to his safety and my sanity.

Just as we were about to go to the emergency room—me with one leg in my sweatpants and Ken already in a pair of khakis—we got the idea that we should call the E.R. to see if they had any tips to try at home. Our local hospital referred us to a medical center hotline in the Kansas City area, and within minutes, Ken was asking the woman on the other end of the phone questions like, "Is Kosher wine okay?"

It turns out that an effective trick involved wine or beer. Lucky for us, we always have many years' supply of that sticky, sweet Manischewitz Passover wine left over from last Passover or maybe the year before that. By the time Ken was using a syringe to aim that wine into my ear, I was singing the Kiddish, the blessing for wine we sing with each of the four glasses during a Passover seder.

Yup, Passover is in the spring, and we were just past the fall High Holidays. For good measure, and because one dose of wine only made the bug drunk, we decided to go for four doses, just like during a seder. Sometimes a moment is so ludicrous all a gal can do is lie on her right side, belting out "Baruch Atah Adonai . . . " at full volume while her husband squirts freezing Kosher wine into her ear. Meanwhile, Ken, drawing on Passover tradition, was reciting, "Why is this night different than other nights?" and pointing out to me that I actually was reclining, something we were supposed to do at the seder but never actually did.

Did you know you can get a little drunk by having wine squirted into your ear repeatedly? Eventually all the wine and singing made the bug give up the ghost. By the time I was in the shower for a long stretch, aiming hot water into my ear to flush it out, I was singing new versions of old Passover songs, including, "Let My Insect Go."

Just before daybreak, I was able to put my head back on my pillow, vividly relieved that there was no fluttering in my ear. But by this point, Ken was wide awake and so was I.

"Why does this happen?" I asked.

"I don't know," he answered. We were lying side by side, starting to make out each other's faces in the low light from dawn. "Is it Sunday?"

I had to think a moment, then told him yes. "Thank god," he said rolling over to try to sleep, but I couldn't, and it turned out he couldn't either. "What do you think is going to happen with the farm?" he asked.

The bug in the ear woke up the bigger (and thank god, metaphoric) one in our minds. "I wish I knew," I answered. "But only if it's good."

Then Miyako leapt on the bed, making both of us jump, before settling down between us and purring us loudly back to sleep.

13

A Twist of Fate

"We've got to sort out the farm," Aunt Wilma said on the phone to us one October night. She had called to find out the latest on my cancer, and after a long catch-up on that, our kids, her kids and grandkids, and great outrage that her assisted living facility in Seattle was considering pulling out the rose garden she tended alone now that Uncle Ron had died, we landed on the subject of the farm.

We had her on speaker phone, near bedtime for us but just a few hours after early dinner for her, and the more she talked, the more the horses of urgency started galloping in us. "What are you thinking?" Ken asked.

"I don't know yet, but surely something can be done. It's not like any of us are getting any younger," she said, laughing. Then she heard our silence on the other end. "But don't you worry. I'm going to look into this so it will be one less thing you have to worry about." Her voice was as soothing as when she cooed lullabies at a screeching Natalie, taking my newborn daughter out of my exhausted arms while I took a nap. Wilma, the middle sister and always the peace-maker, knew how to calm fussy babies as well as agitated adults, and within minutes Natalie was asleep in her arms and I was asleep in an easy chair.

It was no surprise Wilma was trying again to save the farm again. She had been pushing this big rock up the hill for years, encouraging Alice when she tried to buy out her sisters years back, talking to all parties, and at one point even paying an independent appraiser out of her own pocket. Her efforts got more earnest after Opal died in 2006 and gained speed when Alice died in 2018.

"Besides," she added. "It's not like the farm is going anywhere."

Although I got into bed that night as if nothing was wrong, I felt again like that freaked-out young mom holding a distressed baby although I was both characters at once. I was also scared about the limits of what I could or couldn't do. Especially about the farm. Especially about my health.

"Are you going to sleep?" I asked Ken in the dark.

"What do you think?" he answered. We were both shaky with anxiety.

We thrashed about a little, trying to get comfortable, both of our minds rushing through what-if scenarios about this place. No doubt Ken was also thinking what I was, something to the tune of, "But we're just barely out of this cancer nightmare. It's too much." After ten minutes or thirty—trepidation scrambles my concept of time—I asked if he was asleep. He wasn't.

Although it was in the 50s by 1 a.m., we each went outside in our pajamas. A large cloud was traveling over the half-moon. "It's the same sky that's been here for millions of years," Ken said, both of us shivering.

"Except the weather is always on parade," I said.

"Everything is. We're all migrating, even the land." Standing behind me, he wrapped his arms around my chest as we stared into the sky.

He reminded me how this used to be an inland ocean about 300 million years ago, near the equator before this continent drifted north. Waves of glaciers and oceans came and went, leaving behind limestone crinoid fossils, common ocean remnants, and incredibly enough, even two-billion-year-old rocks brought down from the north by glaciers 600,000 years ago. As a former anthropology major, Ken had dug deep into human habitation, and he also had an uncanny ability to remember what he read.

"I'm freezing. Can we go in?" I asked. We went inside and got back into bed.

Back in our warm bed, we talked about the bigger picture of humans here who, according to Ken, lived about 15,000 years ago.

"What about those mounds?" I asked, wrapping myself tighter in the flannel sheets and quilt. By now he was starting to drift off, but he stayed awake long enough to explain that signs of prehistoric humans are more subtle, like the mounds left between 100 BCE and 700 CE by the Kansas City Hopewell, an ancient people who roamed this land.

When I asked him about the native people who lived here before this land was stolen, he was too far gone to answer.

The next afternoon, I reached out to Denise to ask her. My long-time poet friend and the most Kansas person I've ever known, Denise had moved to California a few years before with her husband, Tom, to be closer to family. She explained how the Konza (or Kaw) and Osage hunted and farmed here. As a writer of mixed-blood heritage and a native studies scholar, Denise explained how government interference and the railroad forced south both nations to territorial Oklahoma. From 1854-59, Bleeding Kansas—the bloody border war between Missouri and the Kansas territory—forced bands of Shawnee and Lenape into Oklahoma, also. Only four tribes remained in Kansas.

While I paced the living room catching up with her, I opened the back door to let Shay back in while trying to block Miyako, lest she get out and be picked up by an owl for dinner. By the time I hung up, Ken was home and it was time to throw together a stir-fry and catch up on the day. We also were ready to unpack some of our worry about the farm.

"I'm just too exhausted from cancer," I said as I offered him another slice of whole grain garlic bread.

"Tell me about it," he answered.

I looked into his blue eyes, lightening to a paler blue in the recent years, both of us absorbing more light as people do when they age. After trying out different scenarios, we both got depressed and decided not to talk about what to do about the farm because there was nothing within our hands at the moment to do.

Instead, we ended up on our laptops, researching and sharing information about Bleeding Kansas, a precursor to the Civil War catalyzed by the Kansas-Nebraska act that allowed territories to decide for themselves whether they were slave states (like Missouri) or free states (like Kansas). I read more of the Wikipedia article to him as he hunted for a document he had written a few years about the history of his family on the farm.

Not so coincidentally at the time, Ken reminded me, having found what he was looking for, the New England Emigrant Aid Society sent parties to take claims on land in this county. William Dougal Wells, a 19-year-old from Connecticut who arrived in the society's third party, found southern Douglas County to his liking, enough so that he went back east to fetch his wife, Lovey.

Wells was Ken's great-great grandfather, and because he injured his hand in the Battle of Franklin, one of the first skirmishes of the Civil War, he couldn't fight in the U.S. Army. Instead, he transported gold and other supplies across the country, which led to him luckily being out of town on a momentous day, August 21, 1863. That's when a Confederate guerrilla group led by William Quantrill burned a quarter of our town down and massacred over 150 men and boys, including ones who lived near and on our land.

"So because your grandfather was hurt in the Battle of Franklin, you're here today, and me too?"

"Yeah, that's true. It's all in timing," he said, then asked if we had more garlic bread. Before I could point to the stove, where the leftovers tray was sitting, his phone rang—Daniel was in the throes of finishing his long thesis project, which had turned into a restoration project about the farm, everything circling back to this place. As I cleared the dishes, I thought about how this place has a history of being a healing space, especially for Ken's mother, Alice, who grew up here in poverty and abuse.

Bill Wells himself had come by such abuse honestly. The son of Charles and Minnie, Bill's dad was famous for violently breaking horses. Bill was drawn instead to the glamorous big picture beauty of aviation. He was also attracted to the valedictorian of Redfield, Kansas, Forrest Elizabeth Bulla, whom he married in 1921. Only twenty years old at the time, he surely didn't have any idea what he was getting into, and he ran instead of staying on the farm to learn from place and family how to be a better man.

Alice was a born fighter, shielding her twin Opal and the littler girls with her body while taking on her father's blows. She learned the hard way what she didn't want to pass onto the next generation. Like her sisters, she was labeled "ornery," a word they bandied about with pride for their fierce stubbornness and spirit.

This land gave Alice refuge, as did making a family of her own—
she had regularly told me that having four kids in four-and-a-half years
was the happiest time in her life. Painfully shy, she fell in love with her
shyer driving teacher after she graduated from KU and married William
Lassman, called Gene by his family. Just as Ken's great-great-grandfa-
ther survived Quantrill's raid because of his injury, Gene had a similar
story. Rheumatic fever laid him low in WWII, which kept him from
storming the beaches of Normandy on D-Day with his radio men comrades in the Navy. Most of his class were killed on that tragic day,
another there-but-for-the-grace story that made Ken and our family
possible.

Then again, twists in fate seem to rule the day. When Ken's parents were forced out of their small ranch house on Naismith Street in
Lawrence to make way for a private dorm, Bill Wells offered them a
building site on the land. He was selling Armco steel houses at the time,
able to withstand just about anything, much like his oldest daughter, so
that's what Alice and Gene built with his help.

"My favorite part was when we lived in the basement of the new
house as they were finishing the upstairs. It was all framed in, but there
weren't rooms yet. We also didn't have the furnace installed yet, so we
used the fireplace for heat," Ken told me after he hung up with Daniel.
By then, we were looking at some older writing he did about the history of the farm.

We talked about his mom's love for this land, so deeply ingrained
that she was determined to live here instead of going to any skilled
nursing facility. It wasn't easy. Alice was put on hospice for congestive
heart failure in 2015, not expected to live more than a few weeks. She
kicked that diagnosis to the curb, and although she had lost a lot of
her eyesight and most of her hearing, she was still very much herself,
fiercely determined to die on the farm when it was her time.

Even before Alice died, we whispered to her spirit, vibrant somewhere under the bramble of her growing dementia. Along the long
dying journey, —she was on hospice for three years before they kicked
her off, then she died—she was still attuned to the birds, the breeze,
the view although macular degeneration made it hard for her hard for
see more than blurs of the world. She always knew where home was.

As we finally got to the dishes, I asked Ken when his grandfather do- nated the top sixteen acres of the hill to the county for Wells Overlook Park, named in honor of his father and grandfather. Women and girls, as Ken's sisters and female cousins can attest, didn't count for much to him. "1971," he said. I thought about how I was 11 then, he was 16, and the early '70s seemed as distant as Jupiter.

Lying in the dark while Ken drifted instantly to sleep, I thought about how most of Alice's sisters wanted the land preserved as a family and ecological legacy, but there wasn't unanimity, especially about legal nuances of the trust. Maybe in some universes this would be navigable. But old wounds die hard, especially in pull-yourself-up-by-your-boot- straps and don't-trust-therapists-or-lawyers mindsets, pecking orders and weary resentments, too much water under the bridge and too little listening compounded by time. Like many families, land ownership and how it traverses generations turned into an untenable mess.

I remembered how a decade or more ago, we actually went to ther- apy with the farm with a generous counselor who had us speak to the farm as if it were a living being, which it was. "I see it as a child in the middle of a busy highway, cars and trucks speeding by, and I'm so wor- ried it won't get to the other side," Ken said. Then he started crying.

"Talk to the land," she suggested.

He did. I did. We did. We also talked to a lot of others, including Jerry Jost, the then-director of the Kansas Land Trust, who set up a file back in 2016.

Yet a lot can happen if a person stays put. For years, we stayed and worried. We stayed and freaked out. We stayed and told ourselves we would find a way out of no way. We paced the house at night and often stepped onto the deck, begging for help in finding not just a way to protect this place but how to bring some semblance of healing to the family too.

The wind picked up. I could hear through the dark windows. I told myself this was a sign that help was on the way.

What we didn't know—about the farm, about the cancer—was that this story wasn't a tragedy but a farce when everything seems to be falling apart, life having become an O. Henry story, without the reas- surance in the first act that there would be peace in the kingdom at the end of the third act. In farces, water mains burst, cars stop running for no discernible reason, someone gets a bad diagnosis from x-rays that may or may not have been their own, babies get switched, moony couples end up on the ropes, and bosses force everyone to work right through Christmas with no days off.

But then surprise! The prodigal children return home with a potpie dinner and cream puffs for all, the horrid candidate drops out of the race and humanity is saved, the deadly diagnosis turns out to be a mistake, the right babies find the right parents, and weather and marriages shift to sunshine, daffodils, and freshly-ground coffee.

We didn't know, couldn't know, whether my eye cancer was a tragedy, farce, or something else to be revealed in time. But it was definitely made of mystery, crazy odds, wrong turns that got us home, and especially our relationship with this land, the first thing I saw each morning, the last I looked into the dark of each night.

Both the farm and I were on a road trip without leaving home (quite the contrary). All we had were remnants of maps and gallons of hope and good company. But sometimes those, plus what secret things are set into motion from history and time, turn out to be saving graces. Meanwhile, strap yourself in without leaving home.

14

When Life Reboots You

When life feels out of control, I start counting. I first noticed this habit when I was in labor with Daniel. I was in too much pain to count the seconds of each contraction, but between them, I couldn't stop counting. My mind was immersed in a world of ascending numbers, which made me realize I had been counting anything I encountered throughout the pregnancy, maybe as my way to prepare for the Olympic event of birth.

It was no wonder that many times—especially close to the diagnosis, surgeries, scans, and more tests—I counted days, and when the going got tough, hours. Was counting a way to measure the immeasurable thunderbolt of fear, the stretch of road unfurling around surprise bends, and the drops toward healing that otherwise exist outside time?

On a late November morning, I realized it was 212 days since I heard those dreaded you-have-cancer words. It was 105 days since the first surgery to initiate Operation Tumor Disarmament and 110 days since the second surgery to remove the bolster rockets (radiation implant). But just this morning, I found myself counting forward, not backwards: it was only eighteen days to the four-month anniversary of beginning treatment, and I was closing in on six months since the diagnosis.

Eventually the physical reminders, tiny irritations, and prednisone eye drops, would be as distant as any visceral memory of the pain of contractions. The lessons of all this would come into view over months and years in ways that don't name themselves but surely have to do with what it means to be mortal, the power of love, the mystery of healing, and the conundrum of time. What I mean by the latter is how we get to learn the future is not what it's cracked up to be.

As I moved toward seeing myself as generally okay, out of pain and danger, I stopped counting. Instead, I sat in the house one late afternoon, watching the last few raindrops slide off the gutters and into the flower beds, so overgrown from months of no weeding that it wasn't worth even beginning to find the ground beneath it all. I listened to the soft waves of the crickets as well as a jazzy version of "Jet Song" from *West Side Story*. I felt the ceiling fan's push of air across the hair on my arms.

I stepped onto the damp planks of the back deck, the rain filtering down, and looked into the clouds. Behind them daylight, and behind daylight, stars. So much fire beyond. I thought about what Ken read me from his phone a few days about how the fires in the Amazon, the lungs of the world, were so vast they could be seen from space. I remembered Danny telling me during one of our walks through leaf fall and wind how he'd been crying for the koalas and the Australian eucalyptus forests. The brush fires picked up speed two months before Australia's normal fire danger season. We were watching so much of this in real time on our TVs or computers. Smudges on the screen of the earth.

The world was and still is on fire, and while it may well be worse than ever before, threatening to turn forests into deserts and nations into wastelands, it's also true that the world is always on fire. Over thirty years ago, when I freaked out about the KKK coming to march in our town, Judy, who is also a Zen master, told me how the world was always on fire. She pointed me toward Buddha's Ādittapariyāya Sutta, The Fire Sermon, which he gave to 1,000 monks several months after his enlightenment. What amazed me when I found a translation were these words: "The eye is aflame." All we see is aflame with our desires, aversions, and delusions.

I realized my counting was all three at once, a way to numb myself to all that can't be counted. I could believe I was grappling with reality by counting the CT scans and MRIs for the years to come, but it was just a way to busy the calculator in my mind so it doesn't land in the sloppy swamps of uncertainty. I could count the acres we might or might not be able to buy and multiply the cost by various appraisal estimates, but who knows what's truly possible? We wanted to save this land and my life so much that we could feel it in our teeth, but would counting bring me any closer?

I didn't know. I only knew how to sit here at this moment as the crickets filled the fields and forests. Actually, it is the male crickets amplifying the sound of their front wings rubbed together to draw female crickets.

As autumn fell—wet leaves, crisp air, and all—I realized I was in the middle of a life reboot. I was exhausted more than usual, confused about what eye cancer meant, and reticent about the leftover mini surgeries ahead. I just couldn't get my bearings. But that's what life reboots do: they strip us down to the essentials of staying alive, then re-orient our vision.

All of us get rebooted in our lives, and usually more than once, sometimes happily by falling in love or moving to our forever home, but also through a medical diagnosis, big losses and plunges into grief. Or old dreams diminish to embers. I thought of my friend LaVetta who lost her young adult son, and within four years, her grown daughter. Although LaVetta was out of her mind with pain, she found ways to coach and support others in their grief. I remembered a Turning Point writer who, after surviving cancer and living with lupus and then another cancer diagnosis, decided to go ahead and pursue her PhD to help autistic children.

What we thought was the life plan, the itinerary of our own journey, or the trajectory we were supposed to live could turn out to be a dry husk of a once high-flying insect. Just like when we reboot our computers, we have to shut down the old ways, wait for a new start, and enter some kind of password or otherwise invoke magic words to begin again. Unlike the computer, when the screen comes online again, it doesn't often have all the same icons staring at us, and more to the point, it's not a screen at all but a constantly-in-motion world teeming with life and its opposites.

Sometime that autumn, on the porch just before twilight with Ken, we tried to grapple with the reality that the farm might be rebooted, hopefully for the good. Ken had spoken again to Aunt Wilma, who was moving ahead with the other trustees to hire a lawyer. The scenarios we could spin out of angst and worry, love and hope were cotton-candy light but with none of the sweetness. All we could pick up was the static of our own old tapes.

Then I remembered Valerie's guidance to look at what's really happening right now. We hadn't lost the farm in 12,775 days since we set our intentions on keeping it intact. She also reminded me about how the past can be a good indicator of the future, so not losing the farm for so long boded well.

In this moment, I counted my own inventory of current reality: eleven hedge apples, softball-sized green brains, hanging from the tree I faced, soon heavy enough that we would need to avoid parking our cars under them. Dozens of birds to the west screeched, hawks or blue-jays, loud and angry, or just hungry and determined. Two cats slept beside me, but this was just one point of alignment in a world on fire. Life keeps buzzing its love songs to keep on living.

II

INTERMISSION

WE INTERRUPT YOUR
REGULARLY-SCHEDULED LIFE

15

Beware the Ides of March

"Beware the Ides of March," warned the soothsayer in Shakespeare's *Julius Caesar*. Although he was predicting when Caesar would be stabbed to death in the Roman Senate, the Ides of March has sweeter roots. "Ides" refers to the first new moon in March, usually mid-March in ancient calendars, signifying a new year to celebrate growth and fertility.

Mid-March in Kansas always feels like a new year with all the drama and ambiguity of new beginnings. After the first snowdrop bulbs, a larger-than-life flotilla of blossoms rises in formation. The crocuses come above ground and open into tiny hands of purple or yellow. By mid-March, the magnolias burst into pearly pink boats all over town in such a go-big-or-go-home way that an inevitable hard freeze sends them brown-edged to the ground. Daffodils spring up concurrently with hyacinth, heralding the coming of the lilac and lily-of-the-valley.

Then there's the light returning, lengthening stunted winter days into something else. Birds return and the winter flocks, variety packs of many small and medium-sized birds fighting it out at the feeder, dissolve. All March, the weather wails loud winter storms, then whimpers soft spring breezes before going icy again at such a high volume that the Osage Indians who once inhabited this area called this time of year the Just-Doing-That Moon. If it's 80 degrees and sweltering, it's just doing that. If an ice storm just broke power lines all over town, it's just doing that.

The spring of 2020 seemed especially sweet in its early days to me. The first return of blossom weather brought me up and outside still in the middle of the night, but when I stepped onto the deck early that

March, I felt calmer. Perhaps now I could start to see the whole eye cancer ordeal ebbing to a whisper. I also felt, despite a recently clean CT scan, a strange dread that something was amiss. I chalked it up to old and new farm worry.

The Ides of March in 2020 manifested in a just-doing-that occurrence most of us never imagined: COVID19, followed by a tidal wave of anxiety, closings, fear, and cancellations. The speed of it was stupefying, and my brain struggled to catch up with the foreboding I carried in my digestive tract for weeks beforehand that something very bad had been unleashed. It was enough to make me believe in Pandora, the Goddess of destruction, but then again, the word "pandemic" begins with the same "pan," which means all.

Was it Wednesday, March 13, when we started to realize the pandemic wasn't something happening just elsewhere, although we were charmed by videos of Italians leaning out their balconies, singing dusty folk songs with each other?

That evening, Ken and I set out to hear my favorite novelist, Louise Erdrich, talk about her latest book, her first time coming to Haskell Indian Nations University. All the friends and acquaintances we greeted, all of us holding our new copy of *The Watchman* in hand, laughed about how this was probably our last big outing before the pandemic landed at our doorstep. We were joking. We were freaked out. That night, I couldn't sleep. Something was coming, making distinct clicks on the panic dial as it turned toward us.

By Thursday, I talked with Kelley about how we should send out a reassuring email to the twenty-three people coming to a writing and music workshop that we were leading Saturday. We also decided we should buy some plastic tongs to serve the food and sit further apart. Kim, our assistant for the workshop and also the communications director for the police department, had been in a lot of meetings about what was coming. "Hey, guys, I don't know about moving forward with the workshop," she emailed us. She knew more than we did, but in the rush of emails and our denial, she agreed to show up if we did.

On Friday morning, I woke to a denial hangover. My stomach hurt and head ached as I picked my phone off the night table and started scrolling posts on Facebook and headlines in the *New York Times*. The shaking in the center of my body finally reached my mind. I texted Kelley and within minutes, we were moving our workshop online.

Ken got a call that Sunday, March 15th (the official Ides of March), from his boss, telling him he was on paid leave until this virus blew over. Within an hour Daniel arrived, returning from finishing his master's degree in Wisconsin and planning to live with us for a while. We were soon consumed in helping him carry in boxes of T-shirts and papers from his over-stuffed car, but our conversation was peppered with "Can you believe it?" and "This is crazy."

I went into fight or flight shopper mode, not so much for the toilet paper many were stockpiling but for whatever I imagined we might need for meals for the next few weeks. Maybe a month. At the most. We called Natalie and Forest, made sure they were stocking up on food and meds, and exchanged what to watch on Netflix during our little vacation from life as we knew it. I also started making big crockpots of potato soup and trays of spinach enchiladas, plus maple scones, because desperate times called for desperate cooking.

As we all know, it lasted way more than a month, and the pandemic is still with us in one form or another, but in that initial burst of trouble, we had no such understanding. Neither did we foresee how we'd get used to wearing masks, checking case numbers in the paper, figuring out when to get the vaccine and booster shots for some years to come. We couldn't conceive of the split between anti-vaxxers and people like us who believed in the vaccine, or what ungodly alliances would form in the chaos and polarization.

For months or years, we wouldn't see the insides of movie theaters, sing together, eat non-nonchalantly in restaurants, casually visit each other's homes, or hug people outside of our pods. Articles wrongly declaring that humans wouldn't be hugging other humans anymore popped up as we elbow-bumped each other instead, but humans being humans, they would, at least in my world, launch into even more fervent hugs in a year or so, our masked faces turned away from each other.

In those early days I wondered if the word "pandemic" was overblown, if I was overreacting, if this wouldn't just be a blip of abnormality in our lives. When big things land at the axis of the life we thought we were living, it's impossible to know how far the shock waves will extend. Besides, I was still a little hazy in my cancer recovery, enough that I didn't realize I was still deep in the tunnel, making my way through unexpected turns and drops, none life-threatening, but there, nevertheless.

I also didn't have an inkling that when things fall apart, especially into a locked-up, sprawling chaotic mess, sometimes other things become possible, even when it comes to the farm.

16

Walking Through the New Abnormal

A switch was thrown. The old habits and habitual wanderings and errands were newly sanitized, remote-ized, and curbside-ized. Yep, we even sprayed down our mail, which was relatively easy to do since Ken and Daniel set up a disinfectant schedule and protocol involving spray bottles and washcloths to engage doorknobs and zucchini. We had been somewhat messy people, so the smell of bleach everywhere was disconcerting but hopeful.

That spring was particularly sweet, or maybe we were just noticing more how the birds sang in overlapping harmonies even if some of their songs were about holding onto their territory and driving out invaders. The volunteer peach trees, growing from where we used to have a compost pile, blossomed in their usual aching beauty, although they still wouldn't bear peaches sweet enough to eat. The volume of spring was turned way up, but maybe because I was paying more attention. Yet I was waking up, to paraphrase Rumi, scared and empty.

Everyone started showing up on the street and along the sidewalks in neighborhoods all over town as well as at the Wetlands, a 927-acre preserve, or along the Kaw River trail, or at the Prairie Park Nature Center walkway. Humans, obviously wired to connect with humans and also set to innovation in a crisis, find a way. For many of us, that way was walking.

Waking into a pandemic each day surprised me for months, and some mornings I wondered if this were a dystopian nightmare. It seemed impossible that I or anyone else would acclimate to this collective weight and wait of what ifs and oh nos. But there were counterbalances.

Walking turned out to be our only in-person way of socializing. Ken and I met Forest downtown one April day and weaved through the streets and alleyways of East Lawrence with him, pointing out purple-glitter-spray-painted plastic chairs by trash bins and friendly orange tabbies who didn't know about social distancing. It was an outsider art gallery of a neighborhood of young radicals, old leftists, Latino working-class elders, California gentrifiers, and no shortage of yogis able to do hand stands in their 70s.

Crossing an empty street, I asked Forest, "What's the word for when everything looks one way but it's the opposite?"

"Dissonance? It's 'an anxious tension between two disharmonious elements,'" he answered while reading the definition off his phone.

"Yeah, that's it," I agreed. The world looked the same as we ambled past heartbreakingly beautiful manifestations of spring—tender green just-leafing trees, a gala of daffodils, hyacinths, and even some early scout redbuds showing off like the main attractions they are.

When I met Kris a day later in the wetlands to walk the trails, we talked numbers. The mathematics of people with COVID-19 was exponentially dizzying. More and more people were dying, and medical supplies were running out.

"When will it end?" I asked her as we walked between the prairie on our left, the woods sloping to the slim Wakarusa River to our right.

"I wish I knew," she answered, then we laughed at how we'd been having the same conversation with everyone lately.

"I think somewhere over there was where we had our accident," I said as we turned north to follow the trail the long way round to the bridge. "It's hard to say exactly, though."

"I think I know where it is," she said from the bridge, pointing to a cleft in the river. When I hit black ice driving the kids to school in January of 2001, I learned how much can change in a few seconds. The van dove into the ravine, spinning and flipping at the same time, and throwing Forest, only five at the time, out of his seat. Natalie and I had a struggle climbing out of the upside-down vehicle, but when we did, we found Daniel holding an unconscious Forest on the banks. It was the worst moment of my life.

In short order a medical helicopter took him to Children's Mercy in

Kansas City. Ursula followed the other kids and me in the ambulance to the local hospital, where we were treated and released. Once she drove us to Children's Mercy, she worked on him at his pediatric intensive care bedside for the three days he was in a drug-induced coma. His brain was bleeding in five places and face was broken in three, but a later set of x-rays showed no breaks and bleeding. Ursula's healing work, the medical care, all the prayers from friends around the world, and visitors, coming in two-by-two to see him, plus astonishing grace and extensive luck saved him and us.

Now so many years later, the place where it happened was almost unrecognizable because the state had actually plowed away the road and replanted and sculpted this area into wetlands and prairie, a deal with the devil in exchange for a traffic way linking I-70 and K-10. As the clouds raced east, clearing big swaths of late afternoon blue, the northwest wind picked up.

I dug my hat out of my purse while thinking how the pandemic's impact was a little like what happened to our accident site. It wasn't the place it was anymore and it would never be again. Suddenly, a flood of red-winged blackbirds surged out of the grasses around us, and I wondered if I would one day be able to tell a story of surviving the pandemic just as I tell the story of Forest surviving the accident. Would all these places still be themselves, and what about us?

It was a time when there wasn't enough anti-anxiety medication or slow meditative breaths to lift any aware person out of the vat of uncertainty. With only vague maps and best-guessed timelines, we humans cling to patterns and answers. Yet when I passed people on walks in the wetlands or through various neighborhoods, all of us carefully keeping at least six feet apart, there was a tenderness among strangers. "Hey, how are you doing?" strangers who didn't seem so strange called out, or they'd just smile warmly.

My in-person work—facilitating workshops, meeting coaching clients at a coffee shop, getting together with co-conspirators to cook up collaborative projects—had already been trending toward Zoom and the phone to balance with my recovery. I also had the advantage of having taught remotely at Goddard College for twenty-three years, using Zoom and its creaky predecessors for over a dozen years already. I had learned to turn off my camera and mute myself while turning on the blender to make myself a coffee smoothie to get through a long faculty meeting, and the most common statement of the pandemic—"Please unmute yourself"—was well-worn in my world. But now everything was Zoomified.

My long-time writing workshops at Turning Point shifted from a bi-monthly in-person four-hour retreat to a weekly two-hour Zoom workshop. "You guys see a pandemic and hear about lock-downs and just roll your eyes, right?" I asked them. The twenty or so squares of people with recurring ovarian cancer, M.S., heart disease, or Parkinson's laughed with me. "No big deal to me," a woman with a rare neurological disorder said. "It's not like I go anywhere anyway." For years, I'd been witnessing their ultimate resilience as they struggled with constant pain or a terrifying diagnosis, caring for someone undergoing intensive surgeries or experimental treatments, or trembling alone at home after their beloveds had died.

Time slowed to a crawl, then collapsed in on itself. That second half of March lasted 1,283 days in dread years. But when April—what T.S. Eliot calls the cruelest month—approached, we knew we were in for a far longer, harder month with the virus predicted to peak.

Ken and I made it a habit to walk the fields south of the house, a place we called "the fingers," along the oblong edge of each cedar-lined brome field shaped like a thumb, the pointer finger, and so on until we reached the edge of the pinkie. Then we aimed ourselves diagonally across from the far south end of the land to our house, glowing in the distance. Each step was a question, a plea, a prayer as to what to do and how to do it—about COVID, about the farm, about what dangers might still be churning in my body.

But what did we know about COVID peaks and valleys back then? We speculated that maybe 50,000 Americans would die and ten times that around the world, throwing out numbers as varied as March temperatures. As I write this over four years later, the U.S. recorded over one million deaths and the world over seven million, and that doesn't touch all the COVID-related deaths, long-haul COVID, and damage born of isolation and illness.

It was also the beginning of great acts of love, such as Meg Heriford's commitment to transform her diner, the Ladybird on Massachusetts Street, into a place offering free, hot meals (good ones too) to anyone in need along with pantry boxes and blankets.

People I saw on walks in the wetlands then and for years to come waved and said hello, clearly smiling (visible in their eyes) under their masks. On a three-hour call (don't ask) with AT&T customer assistance, I had a heart-to-heart with a service rep in Indonesia who wanted to make sure, in addition to fixing my account's issue, that I was staying safe and had eaten a good lunch. Tenderness was still afoot.

"You can't get to courage without walking through vulnerability," Brene Brown tells us. We were growing our courage to get out of bed, unsure what bad news would land today and what beloveds of ours (including ourselves) might be threatened, hurt, or just very afraid. Our tentative steps faltered along the paths in the wetlands or down broken sidewalks, trembling like the vulnerable and courageous creatures we are.

We continued our step-by-step dance from the living room to the kitchen, the front door to the backyard, standing still to make meatloaf or bending to pet the dog. Those early days and long nights were not measurable except movie by movie, laundry load by load, walk by walk.

Kris and I waved at each other, six feet apart, in the parking lot at the wetlands, no longer hugging goodbye, and went to the safe havens of our cars. We would walk again, here and on the land around our home where only the trees waved at us, each step reminding us this was just one point in time before another unknown moment.

17

Irises

The turtles returned in the spring with no pandemic threatening them although they had their own challenges of botflies, car wheels, and egg-eating crows. A mask-wearing Ben dropped by, telling me he found Elie Wiesel playing in a mud puddle with Leslie Jones. Using transmitters, he and some of his students were tracking the prodigal turtles above ground and more turtles were ready to be counted in dozens of sites.

Here it was a full year after I was making an appointment to see Dr. Jones in my calendar, not suspecting anything dangerous was happening already. Like last spring, this one was robust with enough rain and heat to make lilac and other blossoming bushes and trees collapse under the weight of millions of tiny flowers.

With the lilacs out, the irises couldn't be far behind. They soon emerged again from underground, falling all over themselves with the weight of their beauty. A banner year, they flung their gorgeousness at us with movie star glamour. For the last fifteen years, I had cut and bundled them carefully in a cacophony of vases in a large box, stuffing bunched-up newspapers in between to keep the vases from breaking on dirt roads. Then I would carefully place the box between Kelley and me as we headed out to the Flint Hills, an area ninety minutes southwest of us, to co-lead Brave Voice, our singing and writing retreat.

This year of cancellations, postponements, mask-making, and stay-at-home directives meant we were not going deep into the Flint Hills to welcome people from across the country to this six-day immersion into writing, singing, art-making, prairie-wandering, and big-sky gazing. I woke up the day we would have gone, went outside in bare feet, and bundled together yellow, brown-maroon, purple-edged white, and dark-blue irises, tossed on some shoes, then drove to Kelley's to leave a vase of irises at her door. The cement landing was damp with last night's rain, but there was enough sun breaking through for some of the worn pebbles in the yard to gleam back at the sky.

Driving home, I thought about how iris petals were almost translucent, their stems prone to complex bends or curves, yet they were remarkably strong flowers. Put a bunch of irises in a vase, and with enough water and care and they can easily last a week or more. Plant an iris bulb, and it will reproduce itself underground, burrowing into the dirt to gather all the nutrients it needs to send up sturdy shoots multiplying over time. Even when the weight of their tops topples them, irises keep opening their buds. They can survive mind-melting summers and subzero winters. They can wind around stones or, as in our front yard, wayward kayaks. In short (although they're tall), they're resilient and brave.

They're also synesthetic creatures. Their scents and shape sing to me, full-throated, putting it all out there. If we could translate them into sound, I think they would sing in a voice that's the love child of Sarah Vaughn and Josh Groban. Their tone is velvety and resonant, occasionally lilting through high notes while also encompassing us in a raw warmth that says home is so much more mysterious and alive than you can imagine.

It also wasn't lost on me that the word "iris" speaks to the flower world and the eye anatomy. My right eye, however, felt even more delicate than this flower that dissolves within a week to a paper shadow of itself. We were all such vulnerable bodies in this world, my tightening throat and lower digestive tract showed me as I went in for another CT scan. Lying on the long hard plastic tray that fed me into the imaging machine, I hoped for nothing remarkable noted in the report we would review with Dr. Soule later that day. Luckily, my wish came true.

Leaving the hospital with Ken after our visit to get the results, I looked toward a stand of yellow irises, leaning away from the wind, some already fallen over. Just like turtles who are far more horizontal and seemingly protected creatures, they tell us, "Fall over but keep going. Dig deep and send up shoots in new directions. Don't be so scared."

18

Impossible Things

As I watched the vase of Pendleton's peonies on my dining room table rush from tight little balls to full-throttle blossoms, I kept thinking of things seemingly impossible to survive: the massive tornado that tunneled through our area last May 28th, my eye cancer diagnosis right before the tornado, and the pandemic topping everything. The peonies were uniformly pink with a scent that could bring people together across political divides to sing in harmony.

Each Saturday, I returned to the farmer's market for the peonies, which burst into full glory whatever the weather and pandemic brought. While the Pendletons' house was still being rebuilt, enough of the greenhouses and out-buildings were repaired, thanks to a wellspring of people with chainsaws and time. The peonies kept producing.

"So you're going to keep going?" I asked John while Karen was wrapping my peonies. They both shrugged, and although we were all wearing masks, I could tell they weren't smiling. They were leaning toward it, they said, and within the months to come, they would climb back into that weather-beaten saddle and ride back into the full life of farming asparagus, peonies, and everything in between. Although exhausted and heartbroken, they would make something good out of the brokenness.

I thought a global pandemic was enough: enough pain, suffering, fear, restriction, uncertainty, and dread. It turned out I was wrong. "I can't breathe," George Floyd said. These were his last words before being murdered in Minneapolis by Derek Chauvin, a white police officer with a track record of violence.

The video of his murder went even more viral than COVID, demonstrating how pervasive the virus of racism is and bringing to the surface more of that pain, suffering, fear, restriction, uncertainty, and terror so many black and brown people have been experiencing all their lives. I understood that I couldn't fully understand what it is to live with the weight of my life threatened for days, years, generations. But I could respect the rage and pain. I could act: march, write, give money, support people acting for the good, and keep educating myself on what it means to be an ally. It wouldn't be enough, but it was one minuscule thing that would be added to thousands, millions of other minuscule things to make a difference.

In June, Ken and I, masked and stepping a little nervously because we were skirting the edge of a crowd, went downtown for the Black Lives Matter march. With all the other masked protestors, we walked past the county courthouse where the police, masked and polite, handed out bottled water as they projected a peaceful presence, even as people passed by with signs that said, "Defund the Police." Across the country, the national guard was called into twenty states while the president, he-who-won't-be-named, ratcheted up the tension with deadly threats. We stayed on the perimeters of the march, listened to the speakers, and marveled at the size of the masked crowd and how everyone seemed to be balancing calm, rage, and determination.

We hadn't been sleeping well, as we worried about our daughter, who lives in Minneapolis. Her neighborhood watch group was on high alert after people in the area saw intruders putting explosives in trash cans. She had one scary weekend with black unmarked vans rumored to be driven by white supremacists moving slowly down her street. Connecting with neighborhood groups, she took her turns staying up all night to be on the watch while also trying to figure out how to hold space for people just a few miles away, who were even more impacted.

In a world of dissonance, there was also this June mood: the wind sweeping up and across the cottonwood tree in that way that told me summer has landed. Three indigo buntings landed on the ground under the bird feeder. Carpenter bees floated above the windows. Moxie, an old border collie and the new rescue dog, fell asleep beside our elderly dog Shay on the deck. The early evening shadows competed with the last long rays of afternoon across the grass, filling with ticks, chiggers, and other summer pests.

Hanging up the phone with Natalie the night after the protest, I walked to the back door to let the dogs out to race in circles yelling at coyotes. The wind picked up, and it was hard to close the door to the big world, where the weather is wild and unpredictable.

"Do you love this world?" Mary Oliver asks in her poem, "Peonies." Yes, I do, so much, but at that moment I was also so afraid of what next year's time of peonies might tell us about the seemingly or absolutely impossible.

19

What Is a Year?

I sat on the deck, watching hummingbirds dive-bomb each other. I was drinking tea in Eureka Springs, Arkansas. I was at the Writers' Colony at Dairy Hollow, a respite for all writers to create unfettered by the obligations of home lives. Two-thirds of the way up a mountain, two side-by-side houses, one a mid-century multi-layered affair and the other an old farmhouse, provide each writer a bedroom, office, and perches outside, like this one.

If you took a town, filled it with winding streets packed with colorful Victorian houses, added some Christmas-light-strewn pterodactyls, rainbow banners, Buddha statues, and homages to the Wicked Witch of the West, then folded that town up and again into some kind of bent cone and put a haunted hotel on top, you'd have Eureka Springs. It's a magic potion of a place flourishing at the hands of lesbian entrepreneurs, redneck motorcycle mamas, and gay artists with a penchant for wind-chimed rose gardens.

I had come here about twenty years ago for a two-week writing retreat, but the guilt from leaving three young kids with Ken, his parents, and sitters back home got to me enough that I bolted after a week. I had longed to come back since then, and when that urge for going seized me, I decided to do just that. We were squarely in the dead-center hurricane of pandemic fear, but I figured it would be safe to isolate in my room, eat the delicious dinners prepared by Jana, the Czechoslovakian cook who could give Martha Stewart a run for her money, and wander up and down the mountain.

Other writers clearly didn't know this or I was just reckless, because within a day of my arrival I was the only writer there. I had lots of company in the wind, birds, and passing-by staff of the colony. A nearly-empty trolley car, driven by a tour guide with a particularly loud microphone, cycled through every thirty minutes reminding me that the empty mid-century house, also owned by the colony, was designed by a Frank Lloyd Wright student.

I propped my computer on my lap, my eyes—one that could see relatively normally and the other living in a soft-edged world of floaters—fixed on the sparrows, jetting from fence ledge to tree branch. We regarded each other while a white-skinned sycamore tree looked on. A whirly-gig—a little thin maple seed swirling unevenly all the way down—landed close enough for me to open up the end and stick it to the tip of my nose, something I did regularly as a kid in Brooklyn.

A year ago, I was positively radioactive and in pain. Now I was jauntily racing my fingers on my keyboard. This tale of two Junes was just a sliver of all the Junes I've lived and hope to live. A year from now, I envisioned a widely-distributed, extremely-effective, and vastly-safe vaccine, and life not going back to the old normal, but opening back up. Maybe I would be back here. Perhaps we would go to restaurants again, peruse bookstores, consider air travel with just a twinge, and think nothing of stopping at a gas station to use the restroom. I imagined meeting friends on the street, talking about how strange it was to have lost so much and so many while also naming what we now know that we couldn't see pre-pandemic.

Of course, I couldn't see in 2020 all the waves to come—the deadly Delta variant, the infectious Omicron winter rampage a year later, many numbered variants beyond that while many of us were getting second or fifth booster shots. I also couldn't know that in just a few months, Myron, a mainstay with his wife Dottie of my childhood, friends with my father before he even met my mother, would get COVID and die quickly. It would be just a little over a year after my brother Barry and I reunited with him and Dottie at the Manalapan Diner, near our old home in New Jersey.

It was beyond my comprehension that my friend Goody, a very young ninety-five, would die from the social and physical side effects of living in a COVID-weary world. Come March of 2021, in the driving cold rain, I will gather with my congregation, chanting and singing the old Jewish prayers in our masks, tears, and steamed-up glasses.

I couldn't know the complications of my upcoming surgery to re-move a cataract and scar tissue from my injured eye. Or how we would arrive home from that surgery to find out that our deal to save the farm had fallen apart. Hell, I couldn't even imagine we would have a real opportunity, set in motion within a few weeks of me returning home from this Eureka Springs visit.

The year 2020 was not lost on me and my injured, recovering eye, going from 20/200 vision before surgery to 20/800 at its worst. Twenty-twenty vision is hindsight, they say, but actually, there are many di-mensions to not seeing in the usual ways or cultivating new sight and insight.

What would we, could we, see and hear in new ways, trusting that with all we lose, there's some compensation of beauty, wisdom, or com-passion even if it's not enough? Encased in wind ruffling the heavy summer leaves while a branch trembled under the weight of a young sparrow, just out of the nest and ready by instinct for what's next, I would write, try to meditate, but fall asleep. Then I'd look up to a deer buck stopped on the leaf-covered ground, staring at me.

Looking out from that writing porch on an Arkansas mountain, I asked the world, what is a year? What is a year from now?

III

THE GATES ARE NEVER CLOSED

20

I Don't Want to Lose the Farm

"The birds are disappearing," Ken told me while pointing to a poster for an upcoming Audubon Society talk. He had just read a Cornell Lab of Ornithology study that found over 53% of grassland bird populations in the U.S. and Canada had vanished.

We had just filled our bellies with the world's best lentil soup and some gyros at Aladdin's where we could eat outside and distant from other humans. This place made sense for dinner. It also made sense because we had a big wish for any willing genies. Last night, Aunt Wilma had called. What she had to say turned all our nothing-can-be-done and best-not-to-disturb-the-sleeping-dragon farm fears on their heads. The lawyer the trust hired, an amiable man named B.J., had talked with all parties to get their perspective, including Ken's and mine some weeks ago. Ken explained how he had managed the farm for decades, and we both shared a laundry list of times we tried to buy or otherwise save this land. It was a long conversation with me doing some New-Jersey-style interruptions to share facts. I was anxious to squeeze into the narrative.

Now we were digesting what Aunt Wilma shared that thrilled and terrified us in equal measure. The plan, if all the trustees agreed, was that the trust would be dissolved, and its beneficiaries would have first dibs on buying the farm at market value, to be independently determined by an appraiser. Ken was the only beneficiary likely to want to buy this land.

The catch? If none of the beneficiaries could meet that market value, then the whole farm would be put up for sale. That's another way of saying that our worst nightmare might come true of the land, including the forty acres around our house, destroyed and developed.

This wasn't just a metaphoric nightmare. When I had cancer #1, I dreamt of giant attack pigs charging into the house. I had deep creases of dream memory filled with images I couldn't forget of crappily-built ranch houses, extending up and down the beloved slopes currently filled with butterfly milkweed, foxes skirting the woods, and fawns playing deer tag across the large expanses. I even dreamt of houses just a few feet from our own, blasting heavy metal music I hated. In awake-land, such expanses of houses were being built within a mile of the farm right now.

As we walked in the swelter of the weather, we talked through the curves ahead. "What if this whole plan doesn't work?" I asked Ken, and before he could answer, I did: "But then we'd be back where we've been for decades, stuck until there's just one of your aunts still alive." He looked at me for a moment, then stared down the street toward the river where, without talking about it, we knew we were going. Both of us were spinning in the realization that we could wait for some unknown quantities of years, then lose the whole farm.

Besides, we told ourselves, the train had left the station, and we had no say to stop it. The longer nothing happened, the higher the cost of real estate, taking the farm further over the horizon of our reach. We already figured the value of the farm had likely exceeded what we could afford, but then maybe we could pay more than we realized.

We started across the bridge, where we stopped half-way to look at the roiling water below and the curve to the east reducing to a vanishing point. It was all too symbolic. What if we re-mortgaged our just-paid-off house and cashed in a hunk of our retirement? Would we have enough to live on in our 80s, and if lucky, beyond that? Right below us, the water rushing over the dam exploded with intensity, spraying mist on us and some sagging spider webs hung on the bridge railing.

My dreams lately were jagged and full of dread, my heart racing as I sat up in bed and asked myself if this disturbance was about my eye and the possibility that some tiny cancer cell had flown the coop and was setting me up for metastatic disease. My body was always too good of a barometer when it came to big things on the horizon, and maybe that was a big thing around us rather than small thing inside me.

"Aunt Wilma was very matter-of-fact," Ken said. We got quiet. "It's like a big ball, and it's rolling."

"You know, we convinced ourselves we couldn't pay more than $3,800 an acre," I reminded him, a number we proposed in our last unsuccessful bid to buy the land. "Maybe we can." I was already making a list of what I would ask our financial advisor, tax accountant, and any banker interested enough to consider a big-ass loan.

We stood on that bridge, shaking each time a heavy truck passed over. Ken was so wedded to this place that I often wondered how he, who grew up forging abiding relationships with butterfly milkweed plants on this hill, would survive if we lost the land. "Hey," I said, "we shouldn't say 'Bought the farm' anymore because it means someone died, and we want to live while saving this place."

"I know he said."

We lived in great risk of losing the land and the great solace of living on the land. All it would take was this delicate possibility of a deal tripping on a pebble, and the whole farm would be up for sale to the highest bidder. We wouldn't be able to stand having our home surrounded by ticky-tacky homes, sprouted overnight as they did in so many nightmares I had over the years.

As we turned to walk back downtown, I did a lot of sloppy math in my head, multiplied and added, playing the numbers game. I knew I was missing vital information to plug into any calculations: what the farm would cost, what we could pull out of savings without blowing our retirement, and how much we could borrow, let alone pay, each month.

Ken and I also returned to our conversation, put on hold since buying the land was put on hold years back, about a conservation easement. Our plan had always been, if we could buy the land, to give the development rights to the Kansas Land Trust in exchange for KLT protecting this land from development in perpetuity. It was a much more complicated legal process than "give the development rights," but essentially, that's what we intended. We could benefit tax-wise from the exchange, we would definitely have some hefty capital gains taxes to pay, but our calling was always to save this place long beyond our lives.

We walked to our car, and late that night out to our back deck to ask the heavens for help, something we started doing again regularly again since Wilma called. Every night. Some mornings. Sometimes one of us but often both. It was showtime but we didn't know if it was curtains for our life in this place, glowing in the on and off echoes of the lightning bugs and the soft summer air hazing everything, or maybe that was my eye.

I felt the warm wind blowing hard and sometimes slowing to a whisper. It seemed to emanate from the trees, pouring from the cores of their trunks, with the clear message that everything was in motion. Although it was dark, I covered my left eye and looked at the skewed layers of darkness with my wounded right eye.

I listened to what this place was saying or holding. The call of a neighbor cat looking for food or sex. A sudden shock of light from a distant neighbor's house. "I don't want to lose the farm," I told all of them. I meant I didn't want to lose my life. I meant this place.

21

The Rube Goldberg Contraption of the Body

Rube Goldberg—no relation, but a girl can dream—is the only person whose name was ever listed in the dictionary as an adjective. The San Francisco cartoonist, inventor, engineer, and reporter, born in 1883 to Jewish parents, grew up drawing nearly 50,000 Goldbergian cartoons of fantastical, complicated improvisations. These included room-sized machines that would take 62 steps to hand the mythical Professor Butts a napkin. Goldberg's legacy lives on in competitions involving pulleys, mazes, chutes, and more for the simplest of tasks.

The body is like a Rube Goldberg invention, or in my case, a Mel and Barbara Goldberg invention. One surprising pinball to the eye zings off an egg, cracking it so that the yolk can drop into a tiny wooden caboose that's now weighted just enough to head across a track, hitting a wall that falls away and sets off a domino cascade of events.

The genetic propensities I inherited for cavities, strengthened by my yearning for chocolate-chip cookies and cream puffs, took on unforeseen dimensions because of all the radiation in my face. Even in the best of circumstances, radiation to the head or neck can wreak havoc on teeth. Add the pandemic to the mix, which made it easier to delay my regular dental visits and heightened the attraction of an apple turnover, and I ended up with news no one wants to hear.

When I finally went to the dentist, I had cavities or worse in all my teeth, some easy to fix, some requiring oral surgery or a specialized dentistry, and many necessitating breaking off hard-won and exceedingly-expensive crowns or implants. Even with insurance, it would be a hefty fee.

While my dentist and I made a vastly unrealistic plan to take care of it all over the next three months, it would turn out to entail a more experienced dentist, two oral surgeons, four years, and many thousands of dollars. The visits were often two or three hours, a variety pack of drilling, scraping, wedging out, or filling in many teeth. I tried to take long breaths through my nose to calm the oceanic white caps rushing in my torso, tips. As there often are in any impossible medication passage, little graces and big humor got me through.

My first dentist's office showed nature videos—armies of penguins pushing themselves and each other over ledges of ice bergs in Antarctica or panoramas of red rock arches—while also blasting '70s rock songs. I tried not to laugh too much because my mouth was open to maximum capacity while a line of ducks slap-footed it across a beach to the Bee Gees' "Stayin' Alive."

It turned out I needed a better dentist with far more experience after most of the teeth my first dentist worked on came down with more cavities. I found a new dentist, a lovely woman from India who would inject the numbing meds without me hardly feeling a thing. By this time, all my teeth needed major work, so I enrolled myself in self-designed dental warrior training. I listened to a new playlist while closing my eyes and traveling into the heart of each song. Taking a Lorazepam ahead of time helped as well as breathing exercises to counterbalance the drilling. This relaxed my jaw when the technician inserted a giant rubber mouth-opener-holder. When it came to oral surgery, I opted for big-gun sedatives, holding the hand of a beautifully tattooed woman with the same birthday as me as I went under.

Maybe it was going to happen anyway years from now or maybe it was just all the dental work, but the drilling hit the buzzer of tinnitus, a constant humming-shushing in my ears. Each dental visit made it worse, yet what could we do?

In the Rube Goldberg falling apart mechanisms of the body, my eye issue bounced into teeth that flipped the switch for ears. My senses were in an uproar. I didn't dare ask if attack monkeys were about to fall from the sky or dog-size locusts would soon sweep across the land.

Clearly, anything was possible, including finding some meaning in a cocoon of white noise. I read up on tinnitus cures only to find out there weren't any. But there are ways to live with it by making friends with inner ear cell damage. First, I learned more about what causes this extremely common ailment that impacts one in seven people. It has a lot to do with damage done over time to cilia, little hair-like nerves that turn sound waves into electrical impulses that the brain assembles into the mind's soundtrack. If damaged, they can't do their work of transcribing the external soundscape, leaving the brain to fill in the void with its own orchestration of buzzes, tones, and other internally-generated sounds.

My ear, nose and throat doc explained it even more clearly: imagine a lake high enough to cover a big rock in it. Then imagine the water level goes down and the rock is exposed. That rock is the sound of your brain working, and what helps prevent weak auditory input from going haywire. "In a sense, experiencing tinnitus is like eavesdropping on your brain talking to yourself although it may not be a conversation you want to hear," says Marc Fagelson, a professor and expert on tinnitus.

So I was hearing the sound of my own mind. If anything told me it was time to start meditating each day, this was it. I chose eighteen minutes a day since the Jewish number eighteen and the letter it signifies—C'hai—mean luck and life. I hooked into old chants from my Sufi dancing days or ongoing Jewish prayers, repeating them in my mind while slowing my breathing. Sometimes I fell asleep. Often I hooked onto thoughts speeding by on the rumination train. But simply by sitting each day, I found myself immersed in the blanket of sound that travels with me always, counter-balanced by listening to crickets or music.

"You'll get used to it," friends told me, and over time, I did and didn't. Sometimes the frequency tuned to a higher, more annoying pitch that startled me. Other times, I experienced tinnitus as a protective shield, a way to keep myself better contained and less apt to jump into what's not mine to obsess over. As someone who struggles to set and hold boundaries because of my worm holes, second-guessing myself, and excessive people-pleasing, maybe being encased in tinnitus was a boon.

It was also clear to me that it would take a Rube Goldberg solution involving multiple layers, buzzers, downward surges, sudden airborne forays, and likely a crazy quilt of bankers, lawyers, family members, seers, and lucky charms. Finding a way to secure the land was obviously—after so many decades of trying so many approaches—a Goldbergian enterprise involving every which way the wind blows through tangled forests and drought-stricken prairies.

But then our collective projects and individual bodies are all Rube Goldberg contraptions, one gift as well as one ailment leading to another, which may require a treatment that sends a napkin across a room meant to gently press on a face. Sometimes the controls go bonkers and the floor ends up covered with broken eggs and tiny cabooses. What to do but get up and start cleaning, knowing that another mishap is in the cards.

The world and the body are made of emergency and waiting, the impossible and the bearable. There's something to listen to in and between all those spaces.

22

Appraising the Bluebirds

Remember the bluebirds, my right eye said in a dream one July, and what it really meant is *remember the lack of bluebirds last winter.* Usually I would see them on the ledge of the deck, arriving in January, ferrying their flash of sky back and forth to the bluebird house we mounted in a ginkgo tree. That blue. That orange. Sure, they can be assholes to other birds, but look at them!

What makes them spectacular has been long misunderstood until recently. According to my friend, ornithologist Rick Prum, and the landmark research he did, they're not blue because they're covered in blue pigment. They're blue because of how the particular cellular structure of their feathers interacts with light, reinforcing, amplifying, and reflecting back blue wavelengths.

In other words, their vibrant color comes from how they're made and how they interact with what's around us, much like us. We also are creatures of where and who we are at once. When it comes to cancer, ingredients are in our bodies all the time. There's a lot of consideration about why some of us activate. We are canaries in the coal mine of environment, heredity, and mystery.

The Turning Point writers constantly show me how we're made in ways that surprise as well as sometimes deeply diminish us. I thought of Lou, one of the workshop participants who I particularly bonded with when an electrical glitch prevented my car from starting after a workshop. By the time we got it sorted it out, we were so hungry that we ended up sharing fries and hot dogs nearby. She was living through a life of Parkinson's, which she developed because of her exposure to Agent Orange as a nurse in Vietnam. But she found a way to let her wings, pitching wildly at times, carry her: She wrote a book called *Vietnam Nurse* and another on living with Parkinson's, which in turn, became life-giving memoirs for many veterans and nurses.

At our best—and sometimes, we're at our best when facing the worst—we can soar into strength and compassion because we're made for it. Humans are also evidently made for greed, stupidity, and laziness, all prone to be turbo-charged by fear, as we know from the evidence around and within us. We can't always see the bluebird when we expect her, but it doesn't mean she's not there.

Sometimes we do see the bluebird, but it's too late. One day while parking my car at the end of our long drive to haul an over-full bag of trash from the trunk into the garbage bin, I was stopped in my tracks by what lay on the gravel. A dead bluebird right at my toes.

I bent down and looked at him, then I picked him up. He looked grayer in death but when I pulled out a wing feather, I saw deep blue: The blue of the emerging sky after hours of thunderstorms, right before sunset when the hue of the sky is richest.

I was late for Dr. Hickman, my new ophthalmologist, to assess whether it was time to do a cataract removal surgery while also clearing out scar tissue shading my right eye's window to the world. The blur of life seeping into this eye had been getting blurrier and more prone to floaters and reality dissolving one thing into another. But the bluebird! I opened my trunk, found a recycled paper bag, gently slipped him in, then put him beside me as I drove.

What did it mean to travel with dead beauty? To ride with a bluebird? I didn't know, but later that evening, Ken and I buried the bird in our yard after I pulled out a few dozen feathers to slip into the CRV's glove compartment. The feathers, along with an orange and white marble, a smooth black stone, pink glass beads, and coins from Mexico—talismans from past adventuress—travel with me.

Seeing the bluebird was a good distraction from what I labeled MFA, Major Farm Anxiety. Yet there were also Major Farm Angels among us, people who shone a light at the possibilities for us realizing our dream. I recently had a long talk with Vaughn, who made a fabled life out of serving in the legislature, farming big acreage, buying and renovating Topeka apartment buildings, and falling in love with Julie.

Vaughn first offered to lend us some of the funds we needed, then suggested we look at what banks could do. He loved our land, having fallen hard for it a few years ago when Ken shared his history and vision of the farm with Vaughn and Julie on our back deck over barbecued chicken and ice cream. But I think it was mostly the tilt of light on the tallgrass, and right on cue, the doe who moved as if she were swimming across a shining pond that grabbed his heart.

Just by him opening the door to potential financing, Ken and I started re-imagining what was possible, something that threw off its training wheels and started speeding down the road once I called several banks and found out that, yes, they were happy to lend us money. Lots of money.

I spent hours filling out loan forms to see just how much we could borrow. One bank looked like a good option, but we would need two loans, one for the land and another one for remortgaging our house. It all hinged on the appraisal, which was happening soon in this late summer heat. Then we'd find out whether we could save this land. I gulped in the quiet, sitting at the kitchen table with multiple tabs open on my computer, including an amortization schedule I visited daily.

To keep things clean and above board, we ended up having no contact with the appraiser, and later found out the appraiser did the deed with a drone and maps rather than setting foot on this farm.

One late afternoon close to 99 degrees Fahrenheit, when we were on the porch with the ceiling fan over us, the floor fan beside us, and lots of iced water, we got the results. The whole farm was $750,000, more than we could afford, but less than our worst nightmare scenario. It was every bit of savings we had, plus our maximum borrowing amount, and more. We'd have to work many more years past when we imagined retiring. But it was—barring the all-too-frequent unforeseeable barriers—do-able, especially if we found someone to buy some of the land.

The next day, I called Victoria, me on my back deck and her on hers. She had walked this land with us for years, talking though how we might protect it, and although she tended toward pessimism about the state of the world, she believed something good would emerge. "I don't know how we're going to pull this off," I said to her. Then I lamented how the issues between Ken's aunts led us to this wildly expensive price tag driven up through years of inertia, fear, and hurt.

"The people who blocked you all these years are wounded themselves," she reminded me, and the wounded are often hurting so much they can't see straight. Victoria and I knew each other's family histories and idiosyncrasies like characters and plot turns in a novel we had been reading together for over thirty years. So I shared with her how I was also shaken by family members who thought we were foolish to even try to do this.

"I believe in Ken and you," she told me, her voice warm and familiar. I was soothed enough by the time we hung up that instead of going back to charts and calculators, I made a tray of spinach enchiladas.

In the vat of what seemed impossible, the numbers could balance out if we found a willing investor to buy about fifty acres. Luckily, one stepped forth, a friend of a friend interested in building his dream home on the west side of the hill. After a few meetings, we shook hands, then got to work on our part.

I spent most of August and early September adding and subtracting, playing the amortization tables like slot machines, calculating how long we'd have to work full-time. We talked money and interest rates, easement restrictions and county regulations into our sleep, which was peppered with little wakings and big anxieties. The What If train came rumbling through many nights, waking one or both of us up to wait for the next sleep train, which was often late to pull into the station.

Losing the farm was a real possibility of unfathomable heartbreak. One night, I sat up in the dark, reached for a Pema Chodron book on my night table, turned on the flashlight in my phone, and opened the book to a random page. I landed on her story about a sign she used to have pinned on her wall that read, "Only to the extent that we expose ourselves over and over to annihilation can that which is indestructible be found in us." I looked out into the charcoal dark of the bedroom while Miyako climbed onto the open book and wrapped herself down in a tight circle, then began purring.

The toll of the cancer, the pandemic, and the buy-the-land-save-the-farm acrobatic show converged that September, careening toward the likeliness of deals falling apart, health threats breaking open, and the coronavirus unleashing itself anew. "Life is death on vacation," Tom Waits once said, all we do to save things, save ourselves, save plans and places were just sandbags piled around our shaky foundations before the big deluge. The farm might slip through our hands, but I had a purring cat nestled into Pema Chodron's words of annihilation. I had this upright body, half warmed in old flannel sheets in this bedroom where I had slept and worried, dreamt and delighted for years of transformations.

I shifted the cat to my side, closed the book and the light, scooted back down careful not to wake Miyako, and gave myself over to the tiny annihilation of sleep. Tomorrow, I would return to the land of tending the body, specifically the wounded animal of my right eye, by way a visit with Dr. Hickman to set the scar and cataract-removal surgery.

Within ten minutes, Dr. Hickman and I were talking about the Bronx hospital where he did his residency in the middle of a vortex of drug deals gone bad and knife fights that didn't end well. He told me he had tricks for getting rid of the scar tissue, and the whole procedure would be over in fifteen minutes unless he ran into trouble, but even then, it would be relatively quick.

The surgery was set for September 16, and if all went well, we might be able to close on the farm a few months later. As some characters in *Almost Famous*, one of my favorite flicks, say over and over, "It's all happening!" Once the old scars were removed. Once the land could see its way clearly.

That night I dreamt of a bear standing outside our bedroom window to the south. She had both paws lifted to her sides, balancing gifts I couldn't see and I didn't know if they were for us. "Not a bear, but a shaman. Bears are shamans and go in and out of two worlds," my friend Denise told me. She explained this was a symbol of power and also, no matter who the gifts were for, generosity.

The week before surgery, I saw another blue bird, this one an indigo bunting, exploding out of its summer red cedar bunch of trees. It was late for him, but here he was, wings propelled in brilliant azure toward our house.

23
Bungie Cords

Years ago, while driving our kids around rural Tennessee on our way to a Smoky Mountains rental cabin, we found ourselves behind a flat-bed truck piled high with dozens of large televisions, strung together with bungie cords. "What could possibly go wrong," Forest had said, pointing to the TVs jiggling and bumping as they went up and down the curves of the mountain road. We couldn't stop laughing. But when you're driving that flatbed, you're not the one laughing.

When it came to the bungie-corded contraption of buying the land, we were the ones driving. Over time, the investor we lined up realized it wasn't as likely he would build a home, but he promised to keep the land intact. By the morning of September 16, right before we drove to the hospital for my cataract and scar tissue removal surgery, he sent an email saying he wanted to talk with us about new ideas for his investment. We knew these words translated into a crop of houses. Either that or he was pulling out.

"Don't," said Ken when I pointed to my computer right before closing it so we could drive to the hospital for our 7:30 a.m. check-in.

"Don't what?"

"Don't even tell me, and don't think about it now." He shut my laptop. I was already more nervous that I thought I should be for this minor surgery on this bright day with refreshing autumn breezes. I was thirsty and of course couldn't drink anything. Now in addition to being a little scared about the surgery, I was a lot scared about the farm.

We found easy parking for the hospital and entered, both of us masked, then went to one waiting room, then another as the hours moved glacially. The Wi-Fi wasn't working, and trying to use our phones as hot spots didn't work either. The 9 a.m. surgery would happen at 11 a.m., then 12:20 p.m., then sometime in the afternoon until someone took mercy on us said we should go home and wait. There were scheduling problems for our surgery room, and they'd call us.

Back home on the porch, I was antsy and thirsty, sneaking tiny sips of contraband water as my nerves climbed more notches. I was also hangry (hungry and angry at once). I sat in my old chair and opened my computer, and there was another email from our investor, this one with an attachment. My stomach dropped—I was sure he was pulling out, and I couldn't even begin imagining alternatives. *Look at kitten videos*, I told myself. *Distract and prepare for surgery. Calm the fuck down.* It took all my self-control not to open the email.

By 4 p.m., we were back at the hospital, me in a gown over my torso and my jeans and tie-dyed socks still on, like a person half in one world and half in another. I chatted up the nurses, but when left by ourselves, I snapped at Ken, who snapped back. Eventually, the calm-the-hell-down drugs began to take me to the land of who-gives-a-fuck, and I was wheeled back to the surgery room.

It was unduly bright, like looking into a tunnel of light, not the best sign, and it was cold too. Dr. Hickman and two young men, jaunty and friendly nurses, joked that this would be easy, apologized for the delays, complained about some insane scheduling gone awry. COVID was wreaking havoc all directions, they explained. One man had a large dragon on his biceps and the other had Dolly Parton on his. I wondered if all the nurses in this town were single-handedly keeping the tattoo shops flush.

My work-horse left eye tried to stay closed without success, so adept as it was at doing the bidding of my hurt eye, which needed to stay open. The overhead light was cold, pressing down into my eye like a metal instrument. I couldn't feel the sharp edges, just the slim weight of ice pushing down. "It will be over soon," I told myself and later found out, repeated aloud over and over to the amusement of the surgical team.

It wasn't over soon. The scar tissue clung on with crafty desperation, and the surgery took closer to an hour. Surgery is always an anesthetized excursion to a realm of wide-open space and vertical blue skies.

The calm of space refreshed me when I was there, flying at 30,000 feet without a plane or destination. Then that space turned into a shrinking bubble, suddenly popped, and I was on the tired shore of beeping machines.

I crashed awake with Dr. Hickman smiling, explaining that it took many more tricks than usual to get out the scar tissue, but it's gone, and after some swelling, we'll see what I can see. I was to come in tomorrow, put in prescribed eye drops, and most of all, rest. Ken and I were relieved, tired, and homeward bound where anything edible sounded good.

By the time we parked, I was too nauseous to eat although I made myself down half a sleeve of saltines. Then, in early evening, I sat at the table on the back deck and opened my laptop to read the investor's email, which included a rendering of a ten-house development. My shaky post-surgical body surged in bitch-slapped hypervigilance. Suddenly, I morphed into *The Beverly Hillbillies'* Granny with her shotgun, I rushed into the house to find Ken.

Soon, Ken and I were on the porch in the dark, me crying, which wasn't good for my post-surgical eye. The removal of the cataract was supposed to improve my vision, and it had but with all the wrong results. We could sell the fifty acres, but then we would lose a big swath of the land as a wildlife corridor and prairie, and what impact would development have on the land we were trying to preserve? We already knew the answer.

I started sneezing, downed some Tylenol and iced water. "This was supposed to solve our problems, not make them worse," I told Ken.

"What the fuck?"

"Yeah, what the fuck!" We yelled this back and forth for a while, pacing and fretting.

We were ready to rail at this reality together. Then we both stopped, overcome by exhaustion and an enlarging sense of defeat. But an idea ran up beside the sadness and took the lead. "Wait, we could try something else. What about Monty and Maria? Would they want to own their own land?" Monty and Maria, who rented land for their trailer from the trust for decades, were fine people who gardened and tended to fruit trees and trails on the other side of the hill. We knew they felt a kinship to this place and wanted to stay.

"What about Hank?" Ken added. Hank, another friend, was the spider expert of Kansas who also had a special place in his heart for snakes. He had asked months ago if he might buy some acres as a research station for easy access to the creepy crawlers and slitherers. I remembered how he and Ken conducted a rattlesnake relocation program some years back for the snakes way too close for comfort to our bedroom windows. People who can re-home rattlers are capable of just about anything.

It happened so fast that some unseen benevolent force must have been orchestrating everything all along. We called Monty and Maria, we called Hank, and everyone said yes. The investor was actually relieved to let go of the promise to buy the land. In less than fifteen hours, the bungie-corded buy-the-land contraption completely changed shape and made it over the mountain.

Had the investor not come forward, we never would have even imagined we could pull off this purchase. That offer gave us scaffolding to get to the height where we could see what was possible. In a sense (and quite fittingly), it was a *Wizard of Oz* moment: Dorothy had the power all along to go home with no magic tricks from the Wizard or Glinda, the good witch of the north. Speaking of which, Maria later told us that line about finding her heart's desire in her backyard came to her in the split second before she said yes to buying the land where she and Monty lived.

"Your eye pressure is too high," Dr. Hickman told me the next morning when I went to his office for a follow-up. "Have you been under any bigger stress than usual?" I tried to answer but something that was both a laugh and a cry escaped my mouth. "You don't want to know," I finally said. He smiled, rolled his eyes, and assured me we would get this pressure down. First, we would try very strong eyedrops, but if they didn't do the trick, he would have to operate on me again to avoid further damaging what damaged vision I had.

As I sat in the examination chair willing the high octane eyedrops to work, I thought about how, if the story of buying the land was a book, this was where we ripped out some pages, then scotch-taped in new coffee-stained ones with fast and sloppy sketches of new drawings. I actually had a notebook open as I thought about this, ready to start jotting down numbers and scenarios. I also was balancing an open laptop on one knee to research other lending options. A sensible person might have closed her computer and notebook, breathed slowly, and surrendered to healing vibes. But I wasn't sensible, my body still shaky and trembling from all the meds flushing through me. My mind was galloping ahead on its mission to save the baby from the burning house.

It took over two hours, but eventually my eye pressure dropped just enough so that I could go home. By then, I had bank applications half-way filled for both a house mortgage and land loan as well. I was also researching another bank's loans that would allow us to roll together the house and land loans into one overwhelming loan.

On the way home from Dr. Hickman's office, I checked my texts at a stoplight and saw two turtles to name. I thought about the pictures Ben sent me of two very gold-flecked guys, each with diamond-patterned shells, and when I got home, I texted him the names of Goldy and Silverado, two old cowboys who had been on cattle drives together for decades. Naming the turtles reminded me of all that was happening right now on the ground despite so much being in the air.

The next days were filled with meetings on our porch or the phone. Monty, Maria, and Hank all agreed to put the whole farm in a conservation easement, protecting their land too, which set off a swirl of meetings with Jerry, the executive director of the Kansas Land Trust, including one on our back deck.

On that October day, he explained, while showing us a multi-colored chart of many extensive steps, how to get from here to there. In short, we would have to buy the whole shebang first, put it in a conservation easement that would protect it from development for perpetuity, then sell them their parcels. But along the way, we would need an extensive land survey of the whole and parts of a three-owner conservation easement, replete with many decisions about boundaries and the "building site envelopes," quickly known to us as BSEs, the only place where a home could be. I offered Jerry another maple scone, and when he said he had enough, I ate it, then another one, trying to numb down my rising worry. Buying the land would be an enormous step. "But wait, there's more!" the universe said as Jerry discussed appraisals, funding, and complex legal descriptions.

I guzzled two glasses of iced tea while listening to Jerry and looking over the materials spread across our metal mesh table. Out of the corner of my right eye, I sensed something in the woods, but when I looked with both eyes, I couldn't see anything. Then, seemingly out of nowhere, hundreds of blackbirds rose from the trees and twisted in a wide river over us. We all looked up, listening to them and feeling the air ruffling around us from their wings.

In between all the meetings, I needed to visit Dr. Hickman daily to check on the eye pressure, which kept flirting with high readings, then settling back down again. I spent a lot of time at his office writing emails to a much-esteemed banker at Rural First, a woman named Linda who said a low interest rate and full approval were likely.

Figuring out the new mosaic of a deal led me to call Dave, our financial advisor, and update him on the story's new wrinkle. "Well, we have over $50,000 in a special account for you to use for a down payment for the land. Remember that?" I didn't, but Dave, who had been listening to our farm dreams for over a decade, did. A farm boy from North Dakota, he often shared old stories of fishing, hunting, getting lost in the woods, or working long days in the fields.

"Should we do this?" I asked Dave. "I mean, you know what our finances are. It's a little shaky."

"Of course you should do this. This has been your dream forever." I could picture Dave, his fair complexion and ultra blond-turning-to-gray-haired self sitting at his desk with three giant computer screens displaying numbers, charts, promises, and risks. I stopped flinching.

But it wasn't just the puzzle of money that had to be in place. We were waiting for all Ken's aunts to sign off on the agreement, which had a December 15th deadline. All but one had signed off, and although rumor had it that she would sign, it wasn't over until it was signed, sealed, and delivered. Until then, we couldn't make an official offer, which led to a Catch-22. Without making an official offer, we couldn't get the needed sales agreement to start processing the loan, which might well delay us from having the funds by the deadline. It was a little like playing save-the-farm Jenga: pull out one piece and hope it all holds together.

For weeks, I woke every day at 4:35 a.m. for forty-five minutes until the next sleep train roared into view and maybe I could hitch a ride back to oblivion. I turned on my side, got uncomfortable, positioned Miyako against me for purring assurance, suddenly got wide awake, paced the back deck in my bare feet even when it was cold and damp, got back in bed and out of bed, got up to pee once I got comfortable again, mind outwitting me from sleep in a sit-com sequence.

We had waited so long. We had bet on the wrong horses, sent letters at inopportune times, and made many missteps. We had prayed to the ancestors for years, as if phoning a friend who could help knock some sense to our heads. Now we were trying to be clear-eyed and right-acting.

After years of talking with the living and the dead, now—on the faith and hope that all would work out—we thanked the ancestors. We adamantly told Bill Wells to clean up the mess he made. We pleaded our case to his mother, Minnie Potts Wells, an Indigenous orphan, who used to play card games and Fisticuffs (and hand-over-hand game) with Ken and his sisters, to their delight.

We reached out to other departed spirits tied to this land. Gene, who grew up in Southeast Kansas and later in the big city of Wichita but saw his work mending fences and mowing the fields as God's work. There were many others too: Ken's cousin Woody (whose real name was Forrest, after his grandmother, and who was a forest ranger) loved this place and understood ecological stewardship. Our dear friend Jerry, dead since 2014, would wander into the south field behind our house, spread his strong arms so that his small frame seemed bigger, and lean back his head in joy while telling the sky, "Thy will be done." We invoked Charles, a pal who died in 2016, and a former Volkswagen mechanic, real estate agent, and Sufi spiritual leader to help us too, especially with the legal end of land ownership.

The ancestors, dead, didn't answer. At least not directly. But the wind tunneled through the talking leaves of Cottonwood Mel, a volunteer tree named for my dead father. Or rain, just a drop or two, came out of nowhere. We took lightning and lightning bugs as good signs., snow or its absence as positive indicators. We listened to and thanked this place for holding us.

A day finally came when I realized that with the cataract and scar tissue gone, although my weakened eyelid kept sloping down to hood my right eye, I could see more. The colors and shapes were fantastically brighter as many others say about cataract surgeries. The green of the cedar was darker, the distinction of the car from the air clearer, and the expanse of the long driveway longer. We were on the right road where the focus sharpened to show all things in motion falling apart and then falling together.

I like to believe that the flatbed of TVs made it to its destination because I've learned to trust in the strength of bungie cords with just enough give to make it up the mountain.

24

Not Going to Boston

Anxiety can make you feel like you're dying even when you're just panicking, as if the word *just* is a slim breath of discomfort. Your chest tightens, breath shortens, throat burns, lower intestines tremble, headaches, mind blanks, and blood pressure shoots up to meet the threatening weather that's real or not. Many of these symptoms could be a heart attack or stroke, so much so that it's sometimes impossible to discern when it's *just* anxiety.

I named the poster child of my anxious crescendos "Boston," epicenter of my worse panic attacks just years after my breast cancer. I was in a very vertical hotel with small rooms and slim windows that only tilted out two inches. It was 2006, and I was there for a conference hosted by a group of writers and health professionals that I overextended myself for at the expense of my health. I had spent wide expanses of computer time trying to navigate roiling waters of the organization's problems. The biggest wave was coming from a challenge that would break the organization beyond repair. Nonprofits are delicate creatures, and although I tried to get people on both sides of this problem to sit down and work out a solution, craziness ensued.

While I was close to three years out from my breast cancer odyssey, I hadn't yet gotten the hang of how to treat my severe chemo-induced acid reflux, which made eating a sandwich a choke-worthy affair. My right heel, dry and prone to cracking, had deep crevices in it and wouldn't heal. I had continual migraines and hot flashes, as my body's thermostat was adjusting to surgical menopause at age 43. I hadn't yet learned what foods sent me to hell in a hand basket (otherwise known as the bathroom). I had rolling sinus infections, my throat hurt, and my insomnia was driving the bus each night. I was also involved in this group for all the wrong reasons: at the request of friends who praised my competence, feeding the people-pleaser in me.

Rooming on a very high floor with my friend Normandi, a poet and Egyptian scholar, the only thing that brought me balance was both of us leaning over the tiny slit of our open window and calling out, "I love you, Blue Men" to the Blue Men theater just beyond the alley we faced. I particularly liked how those words sounded in Normandi's Kentucky accent.

One day, half-way through an all-day board meeting, I realized there was no escaping the truth of what my body was pounding on its drums: I needed to quit. Everything. Right now. I told my friend, who was president of the organization, in the women's room during a meeting break, and although she was generous in her response, I could feel the disappointment in her slim arms when we hugged. I was crying, she was close to tears, and there were over 200 people milling about right out the bathroom door on their way to workshops on the healing power of poetry.

After she left, I gulp-cried for a few minutes, splashed cold water on my face because that's what people did in the movies at such moments, then shot out of the hotel's heavy glass doors to walk Boston. For hours. I wept on street corners while waiting for stoplights to change, trying not to make eye contact with Bostonians, although they seemed to think nothing of a middle-aged weeping woman on the corner. It must happen all the time in that city.

I found delicious clam chowder in an ancient hotel restaurant. I marveled at the golden duck statues in Boston's Public Garden, storied to fame in the book *Make Way for Ducklings,* wondering how to make room for the duckling of my hurting heart. I walked miles although my left heel was bleeding and my head throbbed. I guzzled iced coffee and popped Excedrin well over the recommended limit. I smelled the blooming tulips although I knew they had no scent. I bought a giant chocolate chip cookie at a giant chocolate chip cookie store but couldn't eat more than a bite. I bought Mylanta and downed half the bottle while walking back to the hotel, hiding it in my pocket like a secret flask of whiskey.

I don't remember much of what happened between that wandering day and my arrival back in Kansas, but I do remember that good people hugged me often, told me I would be okay, yet also had a worried look in their eyes as they backed away. I imagine I wasn't speaking very coherently.

What terrified me the most was the sense that I was no longer tethered to reality. I couldn't listen to other humans. I couldn't sleep except in small sips. I couldn't track what time it was, and I had no idea what I should be doing at any given moment. The infinite possibilities of the world overwhelmed me to the point that it was hard to decide whether to take a bath in the narrow hotel tub or fruitlessly lie down and wind through the cable channels. My heart was beating so fast that I was afraid I would never leave this city, never get home again. I was scared I could die.

But I did get home thanks to taxis, airplanes, and Ken picking me up at the airport. Once docked at our house, I still couldn't sleep more than a few hours a night, and I kept crying. "Ken, please do something with me," I said one afternoon. It was still April, and the chiggers weren't out in full force yet, so he picked up a worn turquoise cushion from a lounge chair we found in an alleyway and told me to follow him while I carried the pillow and two blankets he had handed me.

We went deep into the woods just east of our house, a little uphill until he found a clearing big enough for me. He laid down the cushion, had me lie on it, then covered me with blankets while I adjusted my pillow under my aching head. He placed boughs of cedar on my stomach and set a glass of water within reach. The wind rocked the boughs above, and Ken told me to just stay there.

I stayed for a few hours, having given up on trying to fix myself or make sense of the last week. The wind came and went. The mottled clouds drifted across clear blue lakes of clarity and height. A squirrel walked across a branch high up, then ran into a vanishing point. The dog back at our house barked at someone or something. I dozed off and on.

When I got up, it was the beginning of my return to sanity. Since that time, I've been on the lookout for the slippery slope to Boston, one paved with sleeplessness, going against my values, and trashing my health.

Now, so many years later, I was aware of how often my sleep was punctuated by mosquitoes of anxiety. My therapist Valerie had been teaching me about how anxiety races toward a future populated with what-ifs. Sneaky, contagious, and somatic, the only way to keep anxiety on the leash was to take care of this body as best I could through yoga, diet, walks, writing, meditation, and most of all, paying attention, especially to what messes I'm trying to fix that weren't mine to begin with.

No small part of this resilience came from the thirty-five years of trying to save the farm. What were those years? A swirl of late-night conversations on wonky futons or, as we got older and more prosperous, firmer mattresses. Between worn or new flannel sheets. Under quilts I had just finished that eventually became tattered versions of themselves. Sometimes with a new baby sleeping between us as we talked quietly about what could and couldn't be done. Sometimes with Natalie having crept in, a sleepy three-year-old sliding her slim body between our feet and the end of the bed.

Sometimes we were accompanied by a dog, young and nervous because of the thunder, or years later, old and freaked out despite the sedative we gave him at the beginning of the storm. Sometimes it was the next dog, also a lab mix and also thunderstorm-adverse, first young and suave, and now old and rickety.

So many letters were written and never sent or carefully revised a dozen times and sent to no avail. So many letters were received with words in all caps or obscurely written by lawyers that came and went. Files accumulated with maps and proposals, plans and county ordinances, PDFs of aerial views and spreadsheets of what types of acreage compose the whole.

Meetings of Ken's mom and her sisters occurred where nothing happened but hurt and blame, an argument and refusal to talk any more. Rebuffs came at even the idea of mediation. Turned-down offers happened or offers that almost went through but tripped on the final hurdle.

Plus, there were all those awful sentences offered by well-meaning people: "You'll never be able to save the farm." "You need to accept reality." "You need to grow up and let this go." "It's impossible." "You can't afford it and you never will be able to." "You're crazy to keep trying." It seemed impossible in such conversations to convey that there's another kind of wealth that has nothing to do with money, income, interest accrued, and investments paying off.

But other loved ones also buoyed us with words: "I see this happening." "Act as if the land is yours already." "The land wants you to do this." "The ancestors are listening." "You'll figure out a way." "It's a God thing." "Don't give up." And what Valerie kept reminding me: "It's okay not to know how the story ends."

I also kept telling Ken, when we crashed into yet another wall of no, "The only thing stronger than 'no' is not accepting 'no.'"

Now we were pulling into the station of yes, or so we thought. I was better than I was in Boston, having spent years looking more closely at my motives before I made commitments. I had also been laundering my own messes to some success, finding smidgens, then swaths of health and healing, even now with one working eye and the other one at rest but so present.

I woke up too early in early December, slipped my feet in my purple Crocs, and walked out in my nightgown to the deck, frosted enough to glimmer although it needed to be sealed again. "I'm trying," I told the field.

Ken came outside behind me, moving so quietly as he often did that I didn't know he was there until his right hand landed on my left shoulder. We had been up late the night before, me punchy from too much caffeine and angst, and Ken laser-focused on internet-hunting down details of whether a small blue flower was a gentian or something else.

We listened to the wind picking up again.

25

Walking in the Wild, Wild West

"I'm here for my monogram," a well-coiffed silver-haired woman told the receptionist. She was wearing a lemon-yellow crewneck sweater that would look splendid with a monogram on it.

"Yes, your mammogram," the receptionist answered without missing a beat. Obviously, she had heard such variations before, but this is the way of Scan Land, where many, if not all of us, travel to assure ourselves and our doctors that nothing anxious or life-threatening has broken ground or started landscaping itself on our insides. Or we go here to find out how bad the damage is, and whether there's any recourse for repair or just making do in the broken house of the body.

I was there with Kelley and Ken for my quarterly scan to check for micro metastases, which I envisioned as evil bonsai mice ransacking whatever house they could breach. "How many of these have we done so far?" Ken asked me as we sat in the waiting room, me sipping the iodine water necessary for my CT scan.

"You've done too many and exactly what you needed to do," Kelley told me, putting her arm around me. I'd lost count of CT scans, MRIs, PET scans, ultrasounds, all the more specialized eye scans. We had our masks on, each of us filling out forms on clipboards checking off "no" for all COVID-like symptoms. We'd sanitized our hands twice and had our temperatures taken to cross into this land.

I was nervous, mostly about the potential results but also about another CT scan. The body remembers, Ursula had reminded me. This body remembered leaping off the table and fleeing the hospital three years ago during an annual pancreatic cancer screening. On that lovely May morning, anxiety had morphed into a Japanese bullet train revved

up to 190 mph, and there was no staying put, even if just for ten minutes.

But today I had taken a Lorazepam and brought part of the A Team,
three different books, my laptop, my favorite music loaded onto my
phone, and some rehearsed self-talk looping through my brain: *It's just
a scan and can't hurt me, information is power,* and *my body can handle this.*

CT scans involve drinking an oral contrast thick substance, a little
like water but weighing far more, as if drinking it on Jupiter. Then
there's the waiting for the substance to make its way through the body
so that the abdominal planet shows itself in greater contrast. I also
needed blood work to rule out unruly cancer cells on the move.

Today was an unduly long wait, mostly in a small gray room where
I was hooked up to an IV so that I would be good to go as soon as the
looming machine and its technicians were ready for me. It was a tight
space with only one chair and a stool next to the examination table
where I sat cross-legged. When Ken went outside to make a phone call,
I turned to Kelley. "I don't know why I'm so scared."

"Darling," she said raising an eyebrow as if I was describing the
obvious as a mythical creature.

"Everything seems so sedate and calm around scans, and we're sanitized within an inch of our lives, but there's something wild about
them. It's a little like walking with death in the wild, wild west," I told
her, and we suddenly pointed at each other because, like so many such
moments beforehand, we recognized when a song was about to come
over us. Through our many years of co-writing, we got used to calling out "Incoming!" for a new song that was flying toward us even if
we were in the middle of writing something else. We both sensed the
spaceship soaring through the atmosphere to land on the song pad.

We pulled out our notebooks, and within fifteen minutes, we had
the chorus and the first line—"Once the bad news landed"—and we
were off to the races again, calling out words, writing quick versions of
verses. But what really spoke to both of us was this sentence: "Nobody
knows the west/ who hasn't been lost." There's something about the
vast west, perhaps that same western landscape where I was transported
during the PET scan eighteen months earlier, that has always felt close
to the bone. It has a starkness, a clear-skied and clear-eyed way of

seeing the world. A sudden break into wide, open spaces. Or onset of sleety storms seen from one hundred miles away like in Western Kansas. A high lonesome feeling. But in such moments, you hold steady and look up. The gifts of light and perspective are so enormous that it's impossible to fully grasp them.

While walking into the CT room isn't like staring into the big, dark sky of the wild, wild west, there's still that challenge to resist running. "You can learn to see your strength if you stay," we wrote together.

I remember years ago at my oncologist's office seeing two women— one middle-aged and one older, a mother and daughter—walk in the door clutching each other and sobbing. They were sure they were about to hear bad news, and it was hard for them to answer the receptionist's questions. Eventually, they were called back to meet with their doctor, and I was called another direction to meet mine. When I was checking out, they were too, and this time they were crying for a different reason. They had gotten good news, and they were so overcome with relief that they couldn't stop weeping. The receptionist came around her desk to hug them. I had gotten good results too that day, a good day in Scan Land for us all.

Now there was this scan, and in three months, another. Each one felt like a tumble of the dice with mortality, but it's not the scan itself that kills anyone; the scan is just the messenger. *Stay*, I had to keep telling myself, the urge to run so strong, a little like the urge to eat chocolate when I got close to it. Urges come and go and scans too. As long as I kept repeating the same visit with Dr. Soule—"You're fine! All clear."—after each scan, I was grateful, even for running with invisible horses in the wild, wild west of Scan Land.

26

Buying the Farm Without Buying the Farm

Any long journey has its own tune. It has its own hue, pattern, weather, and texture that shifts over time. Ours was consistently unpredictable until the end. It was a medley of prayers, hard rocking backbeats, mournful jazz ballads, and twanged country laments. It was ripped denim left on a fence post until it faded translucent. It was a clear blue sky in one corner, grey-green clouds threatening the center, a suggestion of pink near the horizon, no small amount of thunder and lightning, and surprising snow in May. It was a slip-slide forward, two steps back, a quick grapevine dance, then galloping head-on into apparent walls for days until the closing.

In layman terms, the ending mimicked the whole process with uncertainty until the moment of resolution. Unless we closed by December 15, 2020, the entire deal could dissolve under our feet like the quicksand we joked about as kids as we leaped from the couch to chair without touching the treacherous floor.

Besides the delays caused by an avalanche of people refinancing their homes at the time, there were also strange bureaucratic wormholes that opened up, including a form with certain legalese we should have signed with the bank weeks earlier but neither our banker nor we knew that. Also, our house appraised at an unforeseen low amount, over $50,000 less than even the county tax appraisal. Plus, the national office of our bank was out of sync with the local office, and there were a number of incongruities between the two impacting our eligibility, closing costs, and interest rate.

I spent the first half of December hyperventilating, calling my banker so often that she started answering the phone with a downhearted "Okay, Caryn." I paced the cold deck shivering in my night-gown, pausing to bend down to pet Shay, as I stared into his eyes for reassurance. My mind turned into a Ninja-fighting bureaucratic buster, and I dreamt in multiples of amortization tables.

We were set to go to the title company on Iowa Street to sign a slew of papers for the sale the morning of December 15th, but it took until 4:30 the afternoon of the 14th for all to resolve. The rate got locked at the right numbers, we figured out all the closing disclosure material, and we resolved a bevy of other bureaucratic tangles.

To add to the balancing act, right after we took possession of the farm, we would be crossing Iowa Street to buy a car, my first-ever new one, joking with each other that, heck, if we were borrowing this much money, what was another twenty thousand or so? Over the last year, I had befriended Thom at the Honda dealership as we traded emails looking for what he called "the wild blue unicorn," a Honda CRV with all the bells and whistles a one-eyed-seeing woman needs. It turned out that backing out of most parking spaces requires a person to look over her right shoulder with her right eye taking the lead, which had made for some close calls.

Unfortunately, there was a pandemic-shaped gap in finding reliable nearly-new cars. Further complicating things, I wanted a beautiful blue car. If I was going to spend over $20,000 on a car, it should be a color that made me happy, I reasoned.

One day in early October, Thom called, "Why don't you just buy a new car with no one's miles on it but your own? You can even choose your color."

"There's no way we can afford that."

"Oh, there is. We're having a sale on the 2020s."

We raced over to the dealership and test-drove the car that was to be mine, settled on a price we could swing, moved most of the funding needed from our savings to our checking account, and were ready to file the paperwork. But then I called some finance friends on a whim to ask: would taking out this baby loan upset the big land loan? The short answer: yes. Longer answer: our friends at the dealership held the car for us along with our promise we would go directly there as soon as we closed on the farm.

The night before the closing, we Zoomed Hanukkah with friends. Suzanne, her ex, Bobby, who was also an old friend of mine, and their daughter I had watched grow up. Ken and Daniel bunched up with me at our kitchen table to fit in our Zoom square. Lighting the candles—it was the fifth night of the eight-night holiday—we each shared what light was warming us lately. For Ken and me, it was what seemed forever like an unreachable lantern in the distance: saving this farm.

Now it was the morning of the 15th, a cold and cloudy day. Once at the title company, I pocketed several holiday-wrapped mini-Reese's pieces they had in a bowl before we were escorted to a big wooden table in a small room. They had set up bottled water for each of us, a thick file of papers, and a lovely assistant who worked for the title company. She led us through the "sign here" and "initial there" obstacle course. It was a seemingly ordinary transaction, no trumpets in the distance or fireworks above.

I did all this under my watchful left eye while my right eye, mostly hidden by its closed-shade lid, peeked out approvingly. There was a vaccine just becoming available for COVID, and I told myself we were on the other side of so much danger and dread. These would be more than just temporary lifeboats in the rushing ocean of a life.

It was light and easy, the pen in my hand scribbling out my signature time and again as Ken painted his beautiful cursive one, both of us continually dating everything 12/15/20. At the end, we asked the assistant to take our photo of pretend-signing what we had just signed. The whole thing took less than ten minutes. Then we were out the door again, sitting in our old car, eating some of the Reese's chocolates and giggling. "This is surreal," Ken said.

"It's a miracle," I added, but how that's miracles are. You work and pray, fix a broken drain, give up and keep at it, do another load of laundry, and sometimes, despite the odds and years, dreams align with a certain ordinary moment.

Ken pulled out onto Iowa Street, headed south a block until the car dealership was in sight, and aimed us toward our wild blue unicorn. Soon we were inside, signing more papers, elbow-bumping with our friends who worked there, and we even got to bang the dealership's large gong to celebrate a car sale. Thom brought the new car around, so Bollywood blue and shining that I realized, if this car was a singer, it would be Laura Nyro, because she sang in such a bluesy, vibrant, shimmering way.

Ken and I briefly kissed before I drove Laura Nyro home to where the land surrounding us was, unbelievably, ours. Yes, it was actually the bank's until we paid off the loan, but as I drove down our long, gravel driveway, everything seemed a little different. This was no longer a threatened place in the world. It was safe. The child had crossed the street without getting hit by any tractor trailers. The horses were safe in the barn. The baby was sleeping soundly, and a host of other metaphors were dancing happily. We were all home together, protected and protecting each other in ways that would keep unfolding.

We called Wilma. We called our kids. We ate chicken enchiladas with great aplomb and glee. We washed all the dishes without complaint. We ran out of words that weren't cliches or that we didn't say ten minutes ago.

That night, I fell asleep by 9:30 p.m. in our old flannel sheets and under purple, green, and turquoise quilts I spent years making or mending. The ancestors were at peace, but having gotten in the habit of waking and walking outside in the middle of the night, I woke and went out again, this time with Ken who was also awake.

We stood barefoot on the deck, freezing and grateful, relieved and amazed. All we could say was *Thank you. Thank you, thank you, thank you.*

27

The Prodigal Eye Returns

In *Star Trek*, Captain Kirk can yell, "Scotty, beam me up" with great urgency or casual cheer, and then off he goes. But when he and other crew members land back in the ship after escaping the clutches of attacking lizard-headed creatures or adorably deadly Tribbles (those fur-balls of charm and evil), they often look shaken up, except for Spock obviously.

Every surgery I've been through is akin to being rematerialized in a new place, perhaps just how Captain Kirk or Lieutenant Nyota Uhura are when transferred through particle accelerators without dissolving or exploding in the process. I go into a space transporter device made of anesthesia, then wake up somewhere else—at the least in a recovery room—changed in big or little ways. I've rematerialized over the years without breasts or with a radioactive disk inserted in my eye.

Since my eyelid lift surgery, I've been landing in slo-mo, most of me walking, talking, cleaning out the freezer on a whim or deciding nothing in the fridge is worth eating, except for a spoonful of strawberry jam. The disorientation came from too much light and sight in the newly-opened right eye not meshing with the world. My wider-opened eye wandered like a child, lost and confused in a giant parking lot of some mall.

It started innocently enough a season earlier, Dr. Bukowski met with me in the heart of winter to advise me to think about whether to have this surgery, something that surprised me since it was a given with all the other docs. "Your right eye has compensated for its lack of vision by closing its lid a lot of the time, and there may be a reason for that," he advised. Furthermore, there was a chance—perhaps as much as 25%—that the surgery would result in double or very blurred vision.

Not to worry: if that happened, he could undo the stitch he sewed in a flap of my eyelid in a second surgery. But who wants to go through even a small surgery, then suffer in jumbo-packed visions of everything for weeks before undoing it to get back to where they started?

I did think about it and talk with many people about why I wanted to do this. For one thing, there was the loss of peripheral vision even if the right eye didn't see edges and other precisions. When both were open, even if my right eye was reading in the language of drunk impressionist painters, it still helped expand the reach of what I could see beyond what was point-blank in front of me. What might I gain if my right eye was opened wider?

Mostly there was vanity. It didn't take the people who asked, "Hey, what's up with your eye?" to know my eye looked wonky. Every Zoom session, photo, and video, or glance in the mirror, made me aware of how I looked. I was just like a person I would wonder about. I would wonder if something were wrong with that person's eye? I realized how often I had made ignorant assumptions when talking with people whose eyes wandered, drooped, closed, or twitched. Those judgments were an itchy blanket around me now.

Then I remembered something that came to me once when Ursula, visiting last month from Germany, was talking to me before the pandemic. We were in an office she was borrowing in Kansas City, me lying on a massage table in a pale blue room while she did energy work on me. I wasn't paying attention, and in fact, I fell asleep. Before the treatment began, Ursula had told me to ask for a symbol of what my right eye was, then to speak to that symbol and give it a gift of some kind.

After the treatment ended, sitting in wicker chairs in the corner of that room, I was surprised at what I remembered. I saw my right eye as a delicate being, a small woman walking carefully in her pink kimono with daisies painted carefully on it. She was looking for turtles because she loved them, especially how they could protect themselves in their magical shells.

I saw her sitting on her knees in a garden of irises, tilting her pretty face a little to the left as she looked into the distance. Then she turned and shyly met my eyes. I looked at her, then down at my hands, wondering what I could give her. She and I were both nervous about another eye surgery, even a minor one. She was weary of all the exams, the instructions to look up, and the doctors. She was ashamed of all she couldn't see and how tired she got when being probed by lights and metal instruments, numbed and pressure-measured, stared at by medical professionals in search of what she wasn't. She was also weary of feeling ugly and lidded.

This woman sat back and watched the world, taking it in more than projecting her plans and dreams out into it like I so often did. She could listen like nobody's business. She could look at the one branch of the pin oak shifting slightly in the wind, taking in each leaf it shook loose. She didn't vie for external validation or gaggles of people affirming her place in this world. She wasn't hauling around a heavy backpack of old trauma, only carrying a small porcelain cup, hand-painted with pansies, of green tea. She wasn't me. She was me.

I remembered as a kid being told I had big, beautiful eyes, some saying it was my best feature. My eyes were out of sync with my small face, which made me look like a Jewish anime figure, but I was proud of those big brown eyes (later to turn hazel, then green), so out there in the ta-da! of my being. Just like me, they loved to hang upside down on monkey bars in the park and belt out "People who love people..." or any Rogers and Hammerstein show tune, which did not win me friends when I was six years old.

My eyes opened their attention wide to the giant curious sky of this life, immersed in "why?" and "what next?" and "what if?" Just like me, they learned early that playing it safe and quiet wouldn't serve me in a family where I was often deemed too much or not enough. Or maybe it was more like they knew in the iris of their soul that they needed to defy what might get me ignored, shunned, or beaten so that I could grow the wings I would need and the strength to flap hard.

I was still loud and proud for the most part in my life, but my right eye was in retreat at some off-the-beaten-path unheated cabin surrounded by a few lost cows and a wandering llama. She wasn't ready for visitors or to navigate the journey down the bumpy gravel drive. Wasn't the eyelid lift a way of forcing her? But wouldn't the wide-view and depth perception serve us both?

I told myself that getting my eyelid lifted was a little like wearing a prosthesis after my double mastectomy. I was fine being flat-chested in my cotton nightgown with redbirds all over it at night, but I wanted to boob up when I went out in the world or even settled at my laptop for a day of work at home. Just like I put on my glasses, I put on my breasts, even if the glasses had a more distinct purpose. From a distance, I'm just an ordinary human with a few daily adjustments to look that way.

The surgery was on a mid-April morning in Topeka, somewhere between a beige big-house subdivision and a strip mall selling furniture and donuts. It was chilly, but the explosion of redbud trees and crabapple blossoms even around the sterile medical building buoyed me. Surgery would be short, I was told, just thirty minutes with a half hour on either end for prep and recovery. "You might have some discomfort," Dr. Bukowski told me, but he clarified he meant I might need an Ibuprofen or two or experience pain at a level of two out of ten. I was dubious but hopeful.

The night beforehand, I had written out my intentions at the kitchen table, hurriedly after emailing with Ursula, back in Germany, who said she would be on tap with me that morning, which was late afternoon for her. I saw myself entering into this process willingly, joyfully, and with confidence, clarity, and gratitude. I wrote that I welcomed all parts of the procedure with ease and appreciation, opened the door wide to invite in greater peripheral vision, and intended, as with each surgery, to heal quickly, completely, and easily.

I felt prepared, but all it took was getting out of the car to walk into the doctor's office for my nerves to start jangling like car keys.

"But if you don't do this, you'll always wonder if it might have worked," Anne had told me the day before on a sunny walk with Moxie through tuliptopia in all directions. I told her she was right, but what was up with the tulips? We theorized that last fall, deep in the pandemic, people all over our town—and who knows, maybe all over the world—said, "Fuck this! I'm planting tulips." I had never seen so many before, and I even spied some yards completely ensconced in red, yellow, red-and-yellow-tiger-striped, purple, even black tulips, sometimes well over a thousand where once there was a lawn.

I thought of those tulips planted with abandon as I passed several carefully coiffed squared-off bushes near the building's entrance, not a tulip in sight. Walking into the office of this new medical building, there weren't enough flowers of any kind in my memory to calm my eyes or heart. I checked in and was led to the steel table in back, which made me nervous as well as the quick-paced instructions to hold my arm very still while the nurse searched for a good vein. Part of me was friendly and putting on the puppet show of being happy and calm. Most of me was feeling hostile and considered fleeing to the car. Maybe I'd buy a chocolate donut on the way.

But I liked the doctor and felt a deep sense of trust of him. Soon Dr. Bukowski came bounding over to me. He was younger and more energetic than I remembered. He placed his warm hand on my forearm as he asked me how I was.

"A little nervous," I said while willing myself to take long, deep breaths.

"It's going to be fine," he said, then explained to me that we would soon begin my reunion with fentanyl, Versed, and propofol. But then, they would wake me up so I could open and close my eye enough for him to see where to make the stitches. I knew the surgery was more complex than a few stitches, but to avoid setting the worry dogs free in the nights beforehand, I had avoided reading more about it. Knowing I would be conscious for some of the surgery, even if I couldn't feel anything, it made me want to throw up. But there was nothing in my stomach, I reasoned, so why freak it out about unlikely dry heaving?

"I'm a little anxious, and could you . . . .?"

"No worries, we're going to start the anesthesia right away," he said.

When I asked the anesthesiologist, a square jawed olive-skinned woman with all-business blue eyes if she would say my usual prayer— "You will heal quickly, completely, and easily"—she brushed it off. "You'll only be under for a few minutes." I couldn't help but lean away from her.

I was increasingly not fine, but I did the main thing we all have to do in pre-surgery time: I stayed still. I was wheeled into the surgery room, kicking off the too-hot warm blanket they had placed, at my request, over my torso and legs.

From there, I was someplace else, even when I was back to semi-consciousness with the surgical team all around me. "Open your eye as wide as you can," Dr. Bukowski said. "Good, now stare down at your feet." I willed my eyes down the length of my very quiet body to my toes, somewhere in the beyond.

Then, like all such surgeries, I was in the hazy aftermath of people talking with me, Ken coming in to take notes on what to do if there were issues, then Ken helping me put back on my bra, sweater, and shoes before we tilted out of there toward home.

By afternoon, when the marvelous magic of the numbing medicine wore off, I was okay. I popped an Ibuprofen just to keep the tiny wave of discomfort from turning into pain. I napped, woke and ate popcorn, petted the cat, and talked to people on the phone. It would take some days, probably a week or a month, for my eyes to do their hard-won recalibration dance.

As I started to come out of this, re-materializing as a two-eyed seeing creature, there was a lot to integrate, including the surprise that my right eye was permanently dilated. Hidden mostly under a lid, I hadn't seen this before. This explained why the world was too light-blasted often. The blaring smear of light dovetailed with the lack of definite edges into a halo around everything.

But there was mainly joy here in Mudville, especially as the nausea relented. When I looked in the mirror, both eyes were open and actively learning to track together. One thing that continually dazzled me is how the eyes can reset themselves, our bodies so much more versatile than we imagine.

Later that day, there were turtles to name—Chrysanthemum for a pregnant one, and Clematis from a day I was in a botanical mood, and Sunshine, whom I named when a storm was bearing down, both around and within me.

As the weeks unfolded, I realized I could see a lot more. But it also meant that I was shaken up in new ways, as if some of me was still in one place and the rest in another. During this full landing, I was dizzy, queasy, disoriented, eye-strained, and wiped out, which didn't mesh well with Zoom coaching sessions while also working in Google Docs. I would find out later from the doctor that this nausea and shakiness were normal responses to the equilibrium of two-eyed vision shifting.

There was also deep fatigue, catalyzing me into long, dreamless naps mid-morning or late afternoon. Now my whole body had gone into the right eye's far-flung cabin in a place where no one much visited, and all I wanted to do was sleep between chewing some candied ginger and downing Pepto Bismol. I took activated charcoal capsules for the nausea, which helped. I ate a lot of burnt toast to further counter nausea and watched rom-coms, my right eye tearing up more now that it was so much more open.

I wondered if I was so tired because this was the last of the eye-cancer-related surgeries (at least, that was my prayer and hope). Maybe my stamina was exhausted on the shore after so long being tossed around in the big forces of nature and technology, both healing me and keeping me more hypervigilant that I needed to be anymore.

When I looked in the mirror, I was amazed to see how big my right eye was again, how beautiful. It was a glowing green-and-hazel flower surrounded by a chaos of bruises. Under my eye, there were wave-shaped yellowed and purpled pouches. Above my eye, from the eyelid to the eyebrow, dark rose with black stitches dissolved away slowly. I looked like someone had hit me hard, but the actual eye of the eye was shining and unafraid.

I looked at her in the mirror, and she looked back. She had found her way home to me or vice-versa. The prodigal eye returned to show me how the world was so much bigger than I had imagined.

As I found my way to the other side of the transport, I woke up to tiny nuances and big-ass vistas of this world. I'm reminded of what Antoine de Saint-Exupéry writes in *The Little Prince*. "And now here is my secret, a very simple secret: It is only with the heart that one can see rightly; what is essential is invisible to the eye." True that, but also, what becomes more visible to the eye can show the heart how to see.

28
Pandemic Porches

"You vaccinated?" I asked.

"Yes. You?"

I nodded, then my friend Ardys and I both opened our arms so wide that our hearts had to come out of hiding while we leapt into each other's arms, laughing, pressing ourselves into one another's chests, laughing some more. I could feel Ardys' heart beating into mine. We held on for a long time and the laughter in my body climbed to the edge of tears, so much happiness, and so much to grieve. So much relief that so many of the people I love are alive and well, and so much despair for the ones dead or living with long-term ailments because of COVID.

We were wrapped around each other next to scores of organic chocolate bars at the Community Merc, our long-surviving food co-op in Lawrence. I was there to adopt some of those chocolate bars, plus a few apples and energy bars to take to Eureka Springs, Arkansas, for another stretch of writing as the day is long.

I got the first vaccine in March as I leaned my left arm out my car window while my right eye wept copiously and my left eye just smiled. The second vaccine came two months later, altogether making me feel like I had a magic cape protecting me, at least just a little, from what life can throw at you.

Some hours after hugging Ardys, I unpacked in my Dairy Hollow Writers' Colony suite, and with my computer plugged into an outdoor outlet, I was writing on the porch and open for business. Denise and I call it Po Biz, the work of writing, revising, sending out, filing rejections, and re-sending out poems.

I was also on the seemingly safe porch of my small personal pandemic, happy to be seeing more with my eyesight, still holding to this new vision despite blurred and diminished sight. Cancer is a pebble that lands in the center of a life and ripples out for years to come, changing us in ways that make us more vulnerable but perhaps more courageous and honest too. In a sense many of the treatments for cancer are medical miracles (who knew a gold disk could be sewn into an eye?) even if they will look like barbaric interventions decades from now and leave wounds, breaks, and chasms in us. Just like Leonard Cohen sang in "Anthem," "Ring the bells that still can ring/ forget your perfect offering/ there's a crack, a crack in everything./ That's how the light gets in."

Frightened and anxious, grateful and amazed, I opened my small heart to what the squirrels might be saying in their acrobatic leaps down a dying tree or across an old ravine. The sky clouded over, preparing its wind and rain that would surely come within the hour. I welcomed the peace, grateful to be warm and well-cared-for, in love with all the goodness innate in people also. I was worried about the future, which turned out to be more of a premonition than a worry.

A day later, after an outdoor reading of my writing in the small rock garden next to the library, I got in my car, pulled out of my spot, and drove to where I could turn around. Someone signaled me to roll down my window.

My back right tire was flat, and as I hobbled the car back to the nearby colony, I got a phone text and call at once. The text was from Kelley about how she and her husband were in a car accident that totaled their car. They were fine. The call was from my mom: her sister, my beloved Aunt Rhoda, was in the hospital, likely not going to make it.

Within twenty minutes, AAA was there, and a kind Eureka Springs man with tools and a fix-it attitude pointed out that the tire just had a little puncture. He could repair it on the spot. "Don't worry. This will be easy, and you'll be fine," he told me. I started tearing up, which only made him say more reassuring things that made me start crying.

When I told my writer friends over dinner, choking a little on the words, Jonathan, wearing his "Masculinity is a Trap" T-shirt, reached out and gripped my wrist. Bud, a man in his late 70s who had lost the love of his life a year ago, insisted on washing my dishes, then walked outside with me. When we entered the cooling air of another beautiful Arkansas night, he looked fully into my eyes and said he was there if I needed anything. The heartbroken are the world's experts on heartbreak, especially anticipatory grief.

That night I woke in the dark, loving my Aunt Rhoda, one of my favorite of favorites in the world, remembering how she said, "Oh, Sweetheart" with such tenderness as if whoever she was speaking to was the most precious being on the planet. How excited she and my cousin Renee were when we had a spirited conversation last month on the phone, them in a New Jersey Walmart parking lot where Rhoda was about to go shopping in an actual store for the first time in fourteen months. I was inviting them to a weekend gathering the following November in Florida to celebrate my mother's 80th birthday. All my mom's kids and grandkids would be together in a unique confluence for the first time in over a decade. "Oh, Pussycat, I can't wait to be there and to see you."

"I can't wait to see you too," I said. "And everyone!"

"I love you," she said as she always did in our phone calls, and I told her I loved her too.

Now her kidneys were shutting down. Her blood pressure was in the nether regions. It had all happened so fast. A urinary tract infection made her tired and listless the previous weekend, then she was better, good timing because my mother was visiting. They had a dreamy time with lots of laughter, and Rhoda was even along when Renee drove Mom to the airport for her flight back home. The next day, Renee, calling from work, couldn't reach her mother, so she called 911.

Rhoda died the following afternoon. Her children were in the room saying goodbye, that they loved her, that she could go. I packed up my room and left Dairy Hollow a day early, heading home in a haze of speed and grief to meet up with Ken and fly to New Jersey for the burial. I kept playing beforehand, during, and after the trip the video of Rhoda belting out "Somewhere" (from *West Side Story*) with Renee, a duet they performed at Thanksgiving a few years ago. Her voice was crystal clear as she sang, the remnants of dessert still on the outside table where we listened. It had become a voice I would only hear in my dreams or in old videos from here on. She had forgotten some of the words, but Renee reminded her and also pointed up for when Rhoda needed to climb to a high note.

The day of her burial, we gathered in our serious black clothes, exchanging warm but condolence-polite hugs in the parking lot of the funeral home. As per Jewish tradition, we were heading out to the grave for a short ceremony, luckily enough led by my mom's old rabbi, who also knew and adored Rhoda.

In the hot, breezy enough June, we stood, half-shaded by the temporary canopy set up around the immediate family members. When the rabbi asked if anyone had memories to share, my sister Lauren pointed out how Rhoda didn't just say our names, she sang them, something I hadn't realized before. But it also added to why I loved being in her presence my whole life. My name, and everyone else's, was a song to her.

As per tradition, we passed the shovel, each of us edging in a clump. As with Ken and my family tradition, I knew he would stay and shovel in all the dirt until the grave was full. This was a practice Ken had taken to like prairie grass takes to Kansas soil. I wandered away with the others toward my mother, who was standing by Henry's grave. Henry, her husband for the last twenty years of his life, was a man of great kindness, and we all missed his quiet nods of understanding and his helpfulness toward us at any family event despite how loud and obnoxious we were.

"What's Ken doing?" my mother asked.

"Mom, it's what he always does. He won't leave until the grave is filled."

"He said it would be his honor to fill the grave," Lauren added.

My mother's face changed from incredibility to tenderness that her non-Jewish son-in-law would shovel continuously in the summer heat out of respect for our family and love for Rhoda. We returned to the graveside chairs and sat. Thanks to help from the funeral home, we got another shovel, and my nephews Zachary and Andrew joined in. All these men, two in their 20s and one in his 60s, kept putting their backs into it, lifting hard clumps or pushing in piles of loose dirt. They had long ago taken off their jackets and ties and rolled up their shirt sleeves as they passed around the shovels reverently.

"When they're done with this, they'll need to carve the gravestone, so we might be here for a while," I told my mom, who laughed and cried at the same time.

It was all finished quickly, and within an hour, we were at Rhoda and Renee's garden apartment. There were bagels and lox of course, big fruit trays, the requisite black-and-white cookies, rugulah, and plenty more to nosh. It was a small apartment, so some of us rotated outside, strolling in the sun toward whatever shade we could find among the mature trees planted when this building was first framed.

As the hours went on, I went to my aunt's porch if you could call it that: something between a stoop and a small patio beside her front door with enough room for two folding chairs and a small outdoor grill. Another porch in this pandemic time of losses so big and vast, it was hard to fathom where or when it would end. Yet it brought us together, most of the extended family, for hours of eating, laughing, going through Rhoda's considerable collection of costume jewelry, and telling stories about when she wore this broach or that larger-than-life necklace. There were round silver pendants with abstract reds and blues, resin oval brooches in brown and orange, and Jewish stars in various sizes.

We each got to choose a piece to take home, and I selected a round black pendant with small silver stars on it that I would wear while remembering how Rhoda loved us so much that she sang our names. Leaving Rhoda's, I listened to the birds and all else that couldn't help but sing for their lives.

29

It's a God Thing

It was no surprise that Ken's Aunt Wilma, shortly after the farm was safe and the trust was dissolved, started to dissolve herself. In May of 2021, she died, surrounded by her daughters, singing along to her favorite hymns. She had been happy to be with her grown kids after months of isolation at her assisted living facility.

We had a sense this might happen—her daughters, Ken, and me—and not just because she was ninety-five. Had she not held on, I shudder to imagine what would have happened to this land where she grew up, the middle sister of five strong-willed siblings. She had little choice but to be a peacemaker from a young age. Saving the farm, her daughter Judy reminded me throughout the process, was her God thing, something beyond the realm of human ingenuity although we needed and used all the ingenuity we could get.

I first heard this term from Woody, Ken's cousin, when he was living with terminal lung cancer, a carcinoid that was abnormal—an adjective he emphasized because of how much it resonated with him seeing himself as Abby Normal (riffing off *Young Frankenstein*). We had visited Woody in 2008 and his wife and five Schipperke dogs. They were fast-moving black, small, fur balls with the energy of thousands. Woody had just lost all his hair and was wearing a purple velvet magician hat. Sitting around his kitchen table, almost all of us with a panting dog on our laps, he took off his hat, scratched his bare head, and stopped in the middle of his Robin-Williams-paced patter. "Hey, folks, I know the end of the story, and all I can say is that it's a God thing."

We had, against conventional wisdom (but what else is new?), driven to Fort Collins, Colorado, to see him in January, a month when the

600-plus miles between our house and his were often littered with big or little blizzards. As he spoke, I saw another storm picking up steam, filling the windows with large flakes riding down sideways in the wind.

Woody showed up for people, despite untold distances. I first met him when he drove from the far reaches of Montana to our Kansas wedding, arriving as a total surprise to everyone at the rehearsal dinner. Since then, we had gone the distance for each other. We had embarked upon an ill-fated Amtrak trip with our family, including our newborn Forest (named after Woody, and Ken and Woody's grandmother, Forrest Elizabeth). After the train broke down in Salt Lake City, we ended up renting a car and driving all night, so exhausted that the dark stretches of land seemed like illusions. But we arrived in time for Woody's 9:30 a.m. Idaho wedding.

"A God thing?" I asked quietly.

He nodded, then remembered something that made him leap to his feet and run to the back room. He returned with a small brown-and-blue traveling prayer quilt—a quilt made by Woody, his wife, and his church in San Diego (where they were at the time). They had prayed into each tie they threaded through the center of each square. They sent this to Forest after his accident to help him heal, and when Woody got his cancer diagnosis, Forest sent it back to Woody, who now wrapped it around him like a mini-toga, to complement his hot pink sunglasses while posing like a movie star. That quilt, itself a God thing, would return to us after Woody died.

Now, although Woody was gone, we often thought of him in relationship to our land, which he dearly loved. He often plotted with Ken how he would visit to help us put together a plan for restoring the farm to greater ecological balance. While that didn't happen, our son Daniel's master's thesis did. Daniel spent over five years crafting a prairie restoration plan. Wilma and some of Ken's other aunts were thrilled with the maps, charts, photos, and also their family history embedded in a plan and a dream.

Woody had taught us well the power of showing up, so we didn't blink when it was time to pull out the charge cords and plan a trip to Seattle for Wilma's memorial service on what would have been her ninety-sixth birthday. Ken's sister Karen would go with us, and coming from Manitoba, Linda, flew out too. We all ended up, with lots of other family, the night before the service at Judy and Jim's to eat a dish Wilma and Ron brought back from their travels, one Alice and Gene used to make regularly. It entailed an assembly line of chicken, rice, coconut, pineapple, onions, and other toppings they called Hawaiian or Filipino chicken, depending on who was serving it. We overflowed outdoor couches and chairs, telling stories of Wilma's life as well as tales of how the farm, through her efforts, found its way to the safe shore.

We were also in clear view of another of her legacies. When Wilma and Ron's assisted living center decided to rip out a particularly large rose garden that she and Ron tended over the years, Justin, Wilma's teenage grandson, devoted his summer to relocating seventy rose bushes to his family's backyard. There he created a rose garden in three concentric circles surrounding a gazebo he built with his father Jim.

After dinner, Judy and Jim opened a beautiful oak box where they had plastic baggies of Wilma's ashes as well as some of Ron's, saved from his death four years earlier. We dropped thimbles of those lighter-than-air handfuls of ash on each rose. The Rosa pink and white Double Delight, the deep red Mister Lincoln, the sunset-colored Rainbow's End and the reddish-orange Dolly Parton beamed with fragrance and blossom.

I thought of all the summers Wilma and Ron spent weeks on the farm with Ken's parents, making cherry pie (the women) and mending fences (the men), neither task just metaphoric. When Daniel was born and rushed from the freestanding Topeka Birthing Center to the hospital a few blocks away because he wasn't breathing well on his own, Wilma and Ron posed as my parents. That way, they could join us in the Neonatal ICU, remarking that Daniel, even in an incubator, looked strong and healthy, and all would be fine. I remembered bringing home Natalie three years later when Ron helped us carry the car seat into the house while telling us this was a most fortunate baby. Wilma and Ron, trained through their years as a minister and minister's wife, were both a God thing in our lives and in so many other lives.

I've experienced so many God things in my life before I even had a term for them: Phil, my youth group leader when I was fifteen, who saved me from compounding my trauma through his steady belief in my voice and worth. Ursula working on Forest night and day after his accident to the extent that when the doctors took new images of his head three days later, they said, "It looks like someone switched out the X-rays, like it's not the same kid." Natalie singing "Lullaby in Birdland" in her beautiful alto voice to Alice, who beamed with joy, on the deck in early autumn sunshine just a few months before Alice died. My father holding on for ten days after he could no longer eat or drink until I, just recovering from cancer-related surgery, could arrive. Then, with my hand feeling the pulse on his right knee, he died in a ripple of peace that defied his life. Friends I thought I lost who were just lost themselves and are now back on the other end of the phone laughing with me. So many moments I wept with relief and sadness.

Now a God thing was coming to our farm. A year after Wilma's memorial service, some of her kids and grandkids came for a week of big dinners on our deck and bush-whacking trails in the woods. They would leave behind evidence of their sweat and willingness to brave the chigger-filled forest trails leading from our house to the top of the hill and cleaner borders around fields where cedars had been encroaching. Judy cleaned my kitchen expertly, Jim picked up the tab for a raucous dinner at Free State Brewery, and Jennifer walked her through piles of photos at Karen's house, telling us more about her mother's and father's lives along the way.

We didn't know yet how so many God things would continue on this farm, how we would receive close to $60,000 in funding from the county and from some private donors to cover the landowner costs of the conservation easement. How, three years after buying the land, we would return to the title company one fine June day to sign the papers with the wonderful people from the Kansas Land trust after three and a half years of working together on what KLT board members and staff reminded us was the most complex easement they had ever granted. How, just two months after setting up the easement, we'd returned to the title company with Hank, Monty, and Maria to sign more papers, selling them their land, and how, a few months later, in October of 2024, we would pay off the farm, thanks to a small inheritance that surprisingly came my way.

Even the story itself doesn't know its own ending, but then again, nothing is ending here. It's a continuing circle of land and body. All the plot twists only come into focus in retrospect, including on one momentous and glowing summer evening in 2021.

There and then, Judy, Jim, Judy's sister Jennifer, Ken's sister Karen, and Jim and Judy's kids climbed with us to the top of the old overlook tower at Wells Overlook park to launch Wilma and Ron's ashes into the wind. The hot wind took all we gave it.

Late that night, Ben sent me a photo of a new turtle, an old female. Of course I named her Wilma.

30

"The Gates Are Never Closed"

"But you have to remember, the gates are never closed," Carrie said to us at the closing Yom Kippur services September 16, 2021. It wasn't lost on me that exactly a year earlier, I had eye surgery and both lost and later found a way to save the farm.

. Today our Zoom windows spanned generations and migration patterns across laptops in Kansas, New York City, Pittsburg, North Carolina, Los Angeles, and the Ozarks. All day, from our living rooms or seated at our dining tables, we stood and dovened (chanting prayers while swaying or bowing), sat and sang, read responsively with no one joining our voice but Carrie, our synagogue's president, her Jewish Studies scholar husband Sam, or Rachel, our cantor. This year, I was mostly alone. Daniel and Ken were otherwise occupied, and it was warm and early enough in autumn that I could attend the services outside, aiming my computer away from prevailing winds.

During the Jewish High Holidays, we have a whole lot to say numerous times because we're smitten by the magic of numbers imbedded in our prayers. We're also people of the book, and all the ways you can metaphorize books. The ten Days of Awe spanning Rosh Hashana, the Jewish New Year, and Yom Kippur, the Day of Repentance, start with asking God to inscribe us into the Book of Life. They end with us begging to pass through the gates of prayer in time to be sealed in the Book of Life.

During this time, we are commanded to make amends with anyone we've wronged in the last year, not with a blanket apology for what might have offended anyone, but specific apologies that don't include the words "but" or "if." Ten days ago on Rosh Hashana, Daniel and I stood side by side at the Kaw River throwing crumbs of stale bread into the river as part of the Tashlich ceremony, a word that means "to cast away." We had just finished the short Tashlich prayers, our congregation from ages two to eighty-two, standing in our family bubbles, clutching baggies of old crackers or leftover bread. Now we lined the crooked curves of the riverbanks, speaking our flaws and selfishnesses into the air and throwing one handful of carbs after another into the water.

"I'm sorry for being so impatient with you. I promise to work harder at listening instead of reacting," I told Daniel as I tossed old saltines down the banks.

"I apologize for being so reactive that I argued so much with you when you were just trying to help," he said, throwing a clump of bread.

"I'm sorry for not being kinder with communicating the boundaries I set to take care of myself."

"I'm sorry for my messy boundaries too," he added, both of us clearly products of a lot of therapy sessions, including some hard-won family therapy.

Now on the other side of the Days of Awe, right before Carrie spoke about the gates, and right after Katherine, a long-time member of our community, read the *Book of Jonah,* I shared two poems I read each year about Jonah. The Eeyore of the old testament, Jonah has major avoidance issues. He runs away from warning the people of Ninevah to stop being so evil, something God demands of him in no uncertain terms. But he couldn't outrun God, who cast him off a ship and into the belly of a whale until he promised to do whatever was necessary to get back to dry land.

Once he does the deed and the people of Ninevah change their ways, Jonah is agitated that these people are spared, something he laments while sitting under the cool shade from a tree God provided. The tree then shrivels up and dies. Jonah ends up kvetching to God, who I imagine, in my poem, is really saying, "Once you can have gone so far,/ how can you not let others return?"

What does it mean to return from a hardship, a challenge, a test, a heartbreak, an injury? How can we help others return or at least get out of the way of blocking them from coming back? On that autumn day, we talked about it from Hollywood square-style Zoom boxes, some of us wrapping scarves tighter around us to fend off the chill of the day, in cooler climates, and many in T-shirts under ceiling fans. Bird song, traffic noise, and the hum of the last cicadas traveled the invisible virtual cords among us all. Our voices were more tinny than when we prayed beside each other in person, but we were together while apart.

The pandemic was on our collective minds—all the beloveds we had lost, all the things that had changed or were still changing, all the difference one virus could make. I remembered how Dr. Stein told me cancer would keep changing me, not for months afterwards but over decades. I thought of what Dr. Sandal talked about how our biggest secret is not believing we're actually mortal.

I also thought of this farm, this land, this place where I was lucky enough to be, how continuously it gave me a place to belong. It is a place I'm always returning to. I walk through the gates to what calls from the other side.

I envision old wooden gates, white paint peeling and the latch only working when it lined up just so. It led to an old garden recently spiffed up with red impatiens and pink zinnias between perennial lilies. Iron gates can lead to youthful parks or aging cemeteries. New chain-link gates to amusement parks and especially the open-air Ferris wheel that takes us up to the sweet scent of the ocean in the distance. Gates to colleges full of hope, naivete, yearning, and ecstatic discoveries and fears. Gates to beaches that lead to the end of the world. Gates to prairies that open to a cosmos of grasslands.

There are many gates I worry about: gated communities and the whole notion of making overly-developed land into a fortress for the elite. Gates to prisons when many should be elsewhere finding real paths to rehabilitation. Gates to detention centers, displaced person camps, homeless encampments where people are shoved out of sight and out of reach of food, health care, and warmth. Gates to hell every which way.

But it's the gates of life that I walk toward and through every chance I get. I also drive through them daily, sometimes multiple times when I turn into our driveway, which has an open steel gate we never close.

With others during that Zoom service, our mics largely muted to

avoid chaos, I sang the Shehecheyanu, a prayer thanking God for al-
lowing us to reach this new season. "We ask God to seal us in the Book
of Life, and now that we're nearing the end of Yom Kippur, we cry
out to Hashem to let us through the gates. But you have to remember,
the gates are never closed," Carrie reminded us again. A bell chimed
through my whole body, especially resounding in my tinnitus-encased
buzzing mind. *The gates are never closed.*

We refused to close the gates on saving this land, refused to believe
it was impossible, refused to listen to supposed reason or sense. Instead,
we listened to the sun-bleached grasses in winter light, the fast irides-
cence of the six-lined racerunner lizard, and the wind that also told us
to stay.

The gates may never close for this pandemic or future ones. For
those who died, for the trauma-shaken and heart-broken, for the fis-
sures and craggy breaks in this country and between close friends or
family about the vaccine or virus, and for everyone carrying grief and
love for those they lost. The gates to all this and to the love that remains
are wide open.

We live in a world, a cosmos, and even individual bodies of infinite
transformations. Regeneration is the key that can click open the locks
of danger, illness, even death. I think of all my loved ones long dead or
recently departed, and how something remains.

That night, and the next, and seasons later, I will continue to go
out on the deck each night. I will stand in the dark, half shivering, half
at home in the wind, and listen. Given the odds, who and what isn't a
miracle of life?

The world knows what I want. All my prayers for the same thing:
health and long life, or at least health as long as life grants it. But even
in times of illness, life is granting me this air, this motion of bare or
laden branches, this view that keeps wheeling into time.

Half-circles different directions, and where do I land? Here. Telling
you there's a story to tell—cancer, pandemic, climate change, breakage,
healing, discovery, orange lilies exploding against the house, and so
much more. The story lands me back home where I find ways through,
even in the dark, especially in the dark. It's all here. The gates are never
closed.

Epilogue
WHAT WE'RE HERE FOR

"So is your left eye your bad one?" a friend asks.

I'm startled yet again by this question. "No, it's not bad. It just can't see normally, and it's my right eye. That's the one that had cancer in it."

"Can you see out of it?"

"Yes, but not what you think," I try to explain, usually saying something about how lucky I am to be alive and living on this land that also beat the odds. But when it comes to saving a life or a place, it's standard fare to have to learn how to see as the world and time recalibrate us.

My left eye is my normal eye, taking in everything you'd imagine a normal eye sees, such as the edge of my car bumper where there's a scratch from backing up into a telephone pole one rainy night. It can read faces, tell who's who, and from their gestures or grimaces, discern whether good or bad news is knocking on the door. This eye does all the driving, so when he faces a parallel parking situation that calls upon the right eye to straighten up and fly right, he either sighs and drives on until he finds a parking lot that won't endanger me or studies the back-up camera intently, taking his time.

He's a smart cookie who can read social cues like a rat terrier can ferret out rats. He's canny, sophisticated, at home with a martini or just some over-priced bottled water that's not really from France. He knows how to play poker (and win), make artful sushi that doesn't fall apart when you pick it up, and clean the bathroom to perfection, even if I don't actually do any of those things.

My right eye is nothing like him, at least not anymore. They used to be a married set that cleaned up well for the opera together although they would be the first to tell you that I don't go to the opera or hardly ever dress up. Or maybe they were more like fish-out-of-water pals thrown together in a buddy movie, Richard Pryor meets Charlie Chaplin. Eventually the eyes grew up to join the rest of the body in packing the worn minivan with enough juice boxes, a toddler seat, a baby seat, a pile of board books, and Goldfish crackers before our family headed west.

The eyes worked seamlessly to help Ken set up the tent before realizing we left the little hammer at home and the ground here was hard as rock. They guided my hands to flip pancakes on a grill over an open fire, to the delight of the little kids. Then my eyes led me out, hours later, into the dark of the dark of the Colorado mountain air where I could squat while beholding the crowded lights of the Milky Way.

Now the right eye has gone her own way. Is she bad like some 1960s housewife who finally snaps, trades in the wood-paneled station wagon for an orange Volkswagen, packs it to the gills, leaves the kids at her mother's, and doesn't tell anyone where she's going?

She's not like that at all although it's hard to tell because her museum of realism is closed. In its place, she beholds paintings by the love children of Pablo Picasso, Gertrude Stein, Meredith Monk, Rainer Maria Rilke, Samuel Barber, and Claude Monet. She's sentimental and dreamy, prone to thinking floaters are angels and angles are animals. She sees curled bits of transparent string wound around each other drifting right to the left. She reads the darker places on a face as either a crater or a mouth, a set of black holes or pair of eyes, a chin or slope into infinity.

She can see the bedroom windows, the curtains pulled to the side, the sheen in the window glass made by the overhead light's reflection against the night sky. The cat curled up in a ball on my bed, or is that my brown and white winter hat? Color and shapes, depth and layers, also light spilling—all are bigger and messier for her. So much of what she sees doesn't have edges anymore, reality perhaps more as it is, all-connected. The world is made of soft boundaries.

Without the distinct lines that hold the purple and green quilt as one entity and the off-white wall as another, the dog morphs into the couch. My wedding ring and left hand seem to have always been one vibrant being even if time wrinkles my hand and dulls the ring. When the day ends, where the water of the pond begins or the fur of the kitty extends—all are enmeshed on a cellular level with the air that composes the space between things. Left to her own devices, she sees what she can see.

But it's not just about what she sees or doesn't see. It's so much more than what she sees or doesn't see.

The right eye feels the world in such a tender and vulnerable way that she can hardly stop crying when I put her in charge. She glimpses a television commercial about a credit card company helping a little boy replace his stolen bike, and she tears up at the glory of it. She carefully carries a chipped cup of herbal tea to the backyard, where she sits on a green iron chair, cherishing the way wind leans down the generous branches of summer. She's quiet without agenda in a way I could never be before I met her.

"I am learning to see. I don't know why it is, but everything enters me more deeply and doesn't stop where it once used to. I have an interior that I never knew of," Rilke writes. My right eye is teaching me the limits of the mind's endless hunger to name and categorize things, to know what's what and who's who.

The senses are great compensators, and although it's not as if my hearing improves, much the opposite over time, my being opens wider to music, which the right eye hears in a way her partner never could. When the Indigo Girls, performing in Kansas City, sang the right eye's favorite songs, she cried incessantly, high up in the balcony of the sold-out music hall even though Amy Ray and Emily Saliers were each, from that vantage point, the size of her iris. Her smarter, more able partner didn't even blink, just hoisted himself upward and shook his brow. He's been embarrassed by her a lot lately, but at least he's getting used to her.

She isn't insistent like the eyebrows. She isn't smart like the mouth. She isn't growing larger as the rest of the face recedes like the nose. She doesn't resist the velvety uncertainty of the world. She knows what it is to live in tatters. She understands the softening ground, almost as if it's inhaling the sky one breath at a time all winter until rain can fill in the empty places.

She can see—discern, feel, sense, smell, predict, open her heart to,

hear, even taste something about this life in this place at this moment—
in ways a normal eye can't. Also, sight is always changing, and I realize
this doesn't just apply to my right eye or to me alone.

Along the way, she makes new friends, learns she is stronger than
she ever imagined, and grows courage simply by exercising it. She also
lands on an extra gift, a boon after the journey to the underworld, but
actually, it's not an underworld at all but a wider view of reality.

I open my eyes, grateful for the leaves and gravel underfoot, the
light that rolls beneath the horizon, the horizon itself, and what's up
close and available as air. I'm in the basement on a worn-out maroon
and green floral couch from the 1940s that I scored years ago from a
thrift store. Or I'm perched in a wicker chair on an Arkansas porch,
watching a female cardinal and hummingbird fight for territory. Or
on a plane to Newark, New Jersey, for my aunt Rhoda's funeral at the
height of summer, and months later, on a plane steering east above the
Cascade mountains after the memorial service for Ken's aunt Wilma.
Or on a metal table in a Cat scan room or relaxing on a picnic table in
the Flint Hills of Kansas, watching the sparrows swoop in and out of
their nests. There's so much to see everywhere.

"We don't see things as they are. We see them as we are," Anais Nin
wrote.

How are we made? From stardust and dirt, shit and bones, climate
and climate change, toxins and medicines, the damage and the cure.
Healing is part of us and the earth, made of ordinary and rare time,
weather, and place. Replant what was once a native tallgrass prairie
and let the rotation of the earth for 12,000 years do the rest, whether or
not humans are here to witness it. Find the injury and do something
about it, even if it involves a tiny gold disc with radiative seeds. We're
a tangle of interconnections from the racing threads of synapses across
tree lines and behind eyes, which brings me back to the earth, and more
specifically, to this land where we live, which has its only tumbles and
tangles. Big things to see through small eyes.

Awake and upright, my right eye looks through an opaque and mottled screen. My left eye scrambles up a loose-rocked hill for some solid
ground. How many times can one eye recalibrate to another? How
many times can we forgive each other, or even harder, ourselves? Infinite times or something close to it.

My magic eye. Like all eyes, a kind of nebula in deep space, both a stellar remnant blown to smithereens and a womb for the next round of new stars. A badge of honor. An emblem of survival. A startling new creature able to see beyond sight, but also a sacrifice given gladly to trade for more time.

My eyes and I warily and longingly search for the path in the dark to find my way back whenever I'm lost. This is my life, but it's not quite or really mine. This is the life I get to inhabit, part of the land that inhabits us. We are here to save each other.

Acknowledgments

I am here and healthy thanks to the grace of modern medicine, traditional healing modalities, and a loving circle of friends, family, and community, not to mention sheer good luck.

While there are many loved ones mentioned, there's so much more to say about all those who brought me food, sang to me over the phone, texted me daily, sent beautiful cards or original artwork, and in dozens of other generous ways, carried me through. Thank you with all my heart especially to Ken and our children, Daniel, Natalie, and Forest, as well as to my mother and so many close friends noted throughout the book. I'm also indebted to the medical providers and healers, especially Dr. Sharon Soule, Ursula Gilkeson, Laurie Fickle, and Dr. Komal Desai. So many people brought food, ferried me to and from doctors and healers, and listened to me long into the night when I was frightened, especially Judy Roitman, Anne Underwood, Suzanne Richman, Ravi Bashkar, Dan Bentley, Kat Greene, Rick Frydman, Lisa Harris, Courtney Skeeba, Denise Skeeba, Teri Grunthaner, and surely many others I'm forgetting.

Writing a memoir over four or more years can be a leisurely drive through familiar farmland or a wild roadtrip down many gravel drives that lead to dead ends. Early readers of this book gave me genuine guidance and insight. Bouquets of lilac to Denise Low, Victoria Sherry, Harriet Lerner, Ken Lassman, and Joy Roulier Sawyer. Thank you to all the people who helped me puzzle through how to tell this story, including Kris Hermanson, Kelley Hunt, Kathryn Lorenzen, Jules Flora, and especially Ken Lassman.

Ken and I are indebted for life to the Kansas Land Trust, its staff past and present: Jerry Jost, Kaitlin Stanley, Patti Beedles, Queren King-Orozco, and its board members, particularly Kelly Kindscher and Julie Coleman. Thanks with all our hearts to Hank Guarisco,

Maria Anthony, and Monty Schneck for going on this adventure with us. We also are so appreciative of B.J. Hickert. Then again, none of this would have happened without the miraculous efforts of some members of Ken's family, especially Wilma Johnson.

I'm grateful to and in love with the Writers' Colony at Dairy Hollow in Eureka Springs, Arkansas, where I did the heavy lifting in conceptualizing, writing, and revising this book. Finally, so much gratitude to Mammoth Press and its founders, Denise Low and the late (and great) Tom Weso, as well as to my book design team: the visionary and generous Denise Low, the extraordinary artist Paul Hotvedt, and the proofreader-to-the-stars Jane Hoskinson.

But the place that truly holds my life is the land where we live, continually unfolding and changing as we do the same. I bow to the fields and forest right here.

About the Kansas Land Trust

The Kansas Land Trust works with voluntary landowners to protect prairies, preserving biodiversity, scenic landscapes, and wildlife habitat. Through this work, we conserve native stream banks, reducing flooding and protecting water downstream for recreation and drinking. We strive to expand public access to protected woodlands, streams, and prairies, enriching our connections to nature and each other. KLT protected spaces conserve agricultural lands, generating livelihoods for farm families and resilient local food systems.

The Kansas Land Trust vision grew out of a tragedy. Under the cover of darkness, the Elkins Prairie, a 70-acre prairie near Lawrence, Kansas, was plowed. After years of planning and organizing, KLT worked with the Kansas Legislature to authorize a legal framework to protect natural landscapes for future generations by working with voluntary landowners who value the natural heritage they steward. This led to KLT preserving the Akin Prairie in Douglas County under it's first conservation easement in 1991.

Over the years, KLT has partnered with many supporters, landowners, Fort Riley's Army Compatible Use Buffer program, USDA's Natural Resources Conservation Service, Ducks Unlimited, local governments, and the National Fish and Wildlife Foundation to protect over 40,000 acres. Today our conservation footprint is similar to the size of Topeka spanning across 81 properties in 22 counties.

Included in those 40,000 acres are the 130 acres of Wells Farm, what Caryn Mirriam-Goldberg and Ken Lassman named their land in honor of the family that homesteaded and lived on this land, now – through Caryn and Ken's children, going on six generations. Because of the Kansas Land Trust holding our development rights, this land is protected from development and for a diversity of plant and animal life in perpetuity.

More information: KLT.org

About the Author

Caryn Mirriam-Goldberg, Ph.D., the 2009–13 Kansas Poet Laureate is the author of over two dozen books, including *How Time Moves: New & Selected Poems, Miriam's Well,* a novel; *The Sky Begins At Your Feet:* and *A Memoir on Cancer, Community, and Coming Home to the Body.* Her poetry and prose have been widely published in hundreds of literary magazines and anthologies over the years.

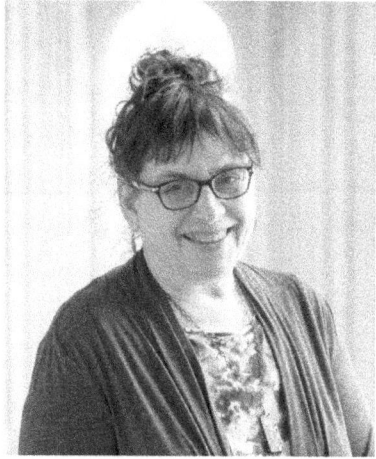

Founder of Transformative Language Arts (writing, music, storytelling, and other word arts for social and personal transformation), Caryn is a beloved writing workshop facilitator and writing coach with over thirty years of experience. She regularly teaches for Lighthouse Writers, Writers.com, the Transformative Language Arts Network as well as offering private classes, all focused on how writing can bring us greater meaning, vitality, connection, and joy. She loves life-giving collaborations: she offers Your Right Livelihood with Kathryn Lorenzen, Brave Voice with Kelley Hunt, and The Art of Facilitation with Joy Roulier Sawyer.

Caryn offers the weekly "Write Where You Are: A Writer's Companion" through her Patreon and her long-running blog, "Everyday Magic."

As elaborated upon in this memoir, she makes her home with ecological writer Ken Lassman south of Lawrence, Kansas where the deer and the wild turkeys roam, a dog and cat keep house, and their adult children frequently visit.

CarynMirriamGoldberg.com

Photo credit: Stephen Locke

www.ingramcontent.com/pod-product-compliance
Lightning Source LLC
Chambersburg PA
CBHW020611270326
41927CB00005B/285